'When life gives you a lemon . . . squeeze it,
mix the juice with 1 ¼ cup of filtered water
and drink twice daily.'

THE LEMON JUICE DIET

THERESA CHEUNG

With a Foreword by Dr. Marilyn Glenville, Ph.D.

St. Martin's Griffin
New York

www.stmartins.com

ISBN-13: 978-0-312-53665-7
ISBN-10: 0-312-53665-8

First published in Great Britain by Vermilion, an imprint of Ebury Publishing,
a Random House company

First U.S, Edition: January 2009

10 9 8 7 6 5 4 3 2 1

Contents

If you suffer from heartburn, kidney or gall-bladder problems, or have a citrus allergy, you are strongly advised to consult your doctor before going on this diet, and you may want to avoid eating lemons or lime peel. Although lemon juice can damage the enamel on your teeth, there are two things you can do to help avoid this: firstly, never brush your teeth straight after drinking lemon juice as this is when most damage can occur and, secondly, keep the lemon juice away from your teeth as much as possible by drinking it through a straw.

Rubbing lemon oil or juice into the skin and drinking lemon juice is not suitable for children under the age of four as their skin and digestive system are not strong enough to handle it; care should also be taken in respect of older children. If you are going to use lemon oil bear in mind that it is highly concentrated and should be used sparingly; a few drops are enough. It should never be applied to skin in undiluted forms. For applications that use lemon peel, always try to buy organic lemons to avoid the harmful chemicals with which commercial lemons are treated. Finally, don't forget that although lemons can prove very effective home remedies for a variety of illnesses by strengthening the immune system, in cases of serious illness you should always consult your doctor first to discuss your medical options.

Acknowledgments

I am extremely grateful to Dr. Marilyn Glenville for reading the manuscript and for writing the foreword, but also for her generous interest and belief in the book.

A big thank you to Clare Hulton for her inspired creative thinking and for helping me see a whole new world in lemons and lemon juice. A heartfelt thank you also to my editor, Julia Kellaway, for her truly inspired direction and insight as well as for her unfailing understanding, help and patience.

Finally, a special tribute to Ray, Robert and Ruth for their love and support as I went into self-imposed exile to complete this project.

Foreword

I have known Theresa for some time now and she has written extensively on many health topics. I am particularly pleased to write a foreword for this book because I know how important it is for people to learn how to lose weight sensibly and healthily.

Some diets make promises like 'lose 5 pounds in a week', and it is all too easy to want those quick results by drastically reducing calories or going on a fad diet. But for healthy weight loss, you can't lose more than one to two pounds a week, and if you are losing more, it is muscle and water. This means that when you go back to your usual way of eating, you will put all that weight back on as fat, and the next diet has to be even stricter. In 2007, the world's largest study of weight loss at the University of California showed that dieting is damaging because of the tendency to regain the weight, and that the yo-yo dieting effect increases the risk of heart attack, stroke and diabetes. The study showed that more than two-thirds of people who go on a diet pile the weight straight back on.

When we talk about losing weight, what we really want is to lose fat. For that fat loss to be permanent you need to lose it slowly, and by following the recommendations in this book you will do so easily and healthily. And not only will you lose weight, you will improve your digestion too because you are not just what you eat, but also what you digest and absorb. The guidelines in this book will, in addition, help improve your general health and by getting your blood sugar in balance you may find that other symptoms will disappear such as mood swings, irritability, depression, fatigue, lack of sex drive, insomnia and PMS.

Dr. Marilyn Glenville, Ph.D.
Nutritionist, President of the Food and Health Forum of the Royal Society of Medicine (U.K.), and author of *Fat Around the Middle*
www.marilynglenville.com

Introduction: Lemon Twist

If you've picked up this book thinking it's a lemon juice detox for drastic weight loss, you'll be disappointed. A common myth is that you can lose a significant amount of weight by detoxing or starving yourself for days on end with juice and water as your only sustenance. Such detox diets are always based on *fantasy* instead of *science*. Most importantly, any eating plan that does not supply an average of 1,200 calories a day is not safe or supportive of optimal health or long-term weight loss. It can lead to intense and unpleasant side effects, including stomach pain, diarrhea, dizziness, nausea, vomiting, fever, headaches, blurred vision and fatigue.

Scientists are also confirming what most nutritionists have known all along: severely restricting your food intake, or cutting out certain food groups, to lose weight simply *doesn't work* in the long term. Putting yourself on a fad diet, a juice fast or only sipping hot water with lemon for days on end will just slow down your metabolism (fat burning), decrease your blood sugar levels and make you feel moody, tired and sluggish.

In addition, fad diets simply aren't sustainable because they are so restrictive. Any weight that you lose will mostly be water, and as soon as you eat normally again you will put all the weight back on. You will also be susceptible to saggy skin where you've lost muscle and to gaining a few extra pounds because your metabolism has slowed down with the dieting. And fad diets that cut out certain food groups don't give you the nutrients you need to keep your skin smooth, your belly firm and your breath fresh. Finally, if you cut down on essential nutrients you increase your risk of heart disease, stroke, diabetes, osteoporosis and even cancer.

WHY THE LEMON JUICE DIET IS DIFFERENT

So, if dieting is a waste of time and energy, why is the Lemon Juice Diet any different? As we have seen, there is no science behind the claim that fasting and detox in the long term can help you lose weight safely and effectively. However, there is scientific evidence for the benefits of short-term nutritional detoxification, when supervised properly. A short fast – for no more than one or two days – can give your digestion, absorption and liver function a nutritional restart. In other words, it can boost your body's natural detoxification process.

You may not realize it but your body is constantly detoxing itself naturally. Your digestive system is pretty efficient at cleansing itself and ridding your body of toxins. The liver is the major detoxification organ in the body, and the kidneys are the major filtration system. Fasting doesn't purify your body of toxins; these organs do. If your diet is poor or you aren't giving your in-house detoxification system the nutrients it needs to function properly, this can lead to poor digestion and toxic build-up. In this case, a one-day semi-fast can help clear those toxins and replenish lost nutrients which your body needs to burn fat.

It's the strong emphasis on digestion that makes the Lemon Juice Diet different. There is nothing more important to your health and your weight than the function of your digestive system. If your digestion is healthy, 'good-for-you' nutrients are broken down and digested and 'not-so-good-for-you' substances discarded. However, if your digestive system isn't functioning optimally, it doesn't matter how many so-called superfoods you eat, you won't be getting the nutrients your body needs to be healthy, to detox naturally and to rev up your metabolism.

When it comes to boosting the body's digestive and detox systems, lemon is a natural powerhouse with an energizing tangy flavor. It is therefore exactly the right food not only to kick-start your weight loss but also to help you keep the weight off for good. Its vitamin C content also gives it powerful immune-boosting properties. It's not surprising, therefore, that nutritionists tend to recommend it as the first drink of the morning.

To lose weight healthily you need to eat the most nutritious foods possible to boost your metabolism, digestion and your body's natural detoxification processes. The Lemon Juice Diet is not a 'diet' as such but a simple healthy-eating plan based around digestion-boosting foods, such as lemon, that will encourage your body to detox naturally and provide you with the essential nutrients for radiant skin, strong bones and boundless energy. It's a diet built to last you a lifetime. Your health will improve and you will lose weight. Best of all, you'll find it so effective and simple to follow that you'll never pick up another diet book.

HOW TO USE THIS BOOK

If you've got weight to lose, previous diets may not have succeeded because your digestion is poor and, as a result, your metabolism is sluggish. Each chapter in this book is designed to help you tune up your digestion so you can reap the rewards in terms of extra health and energy while the pounds melt away.

Chapter 1 explains the weight-loss benefits of lemons. In Chapter 2 you'll be encouraged to begin your diet with a one-day lemon juice detox. This isn't what is commonly known as a 'detox'. Rather, it is a nutritionally sound, step-by-step, healthy-eating day to boost your digestion, eliminate toxins and kick-start your weight loss. Chapter 3 helps you get started with shopping and cooking guidelines and some helpful motivational advice. But if you want to jump right in you can go straight to Chapter 4, which sets out clearly and simply the seven Lemon Juice Diet principles, encouraging you to implement each principle over a seven-day period. In this way you can begin to feel the energy-boosting benefits of the Lemon Juice Diet within seven days and the weight-loss benefits within 14 days. Chapter 5 suggests menu plans that you can use once you have worked through the seven principles.

Chapter 6 will give you valuable tips on buying, cooking, and storing lemons, as well as providing a selection of mouth-watering lemon-based recipes to help boost weight loss. Chapter 7 is your exercise program. Gentle exercise is a great way to rev up your metabolism because the more you move, the more calories your body needs. Also, if you're active you build up muscle, and the more muscle you have, the more calories you burn. If you haven't exercised for a while or hate exercising, don't panic. You don't have to join a gym or jog for miles every day on the Lemon Juice Diet; this chapter will show you how simple and fun lifestyle changes can make a huge difference to your waistline. If you suffer from food cravings or lack of willpower, Chapter 8 is packed with motivational advice and suggestions to help you get back on track. Chapter 9 is an A–Z list of common ailments that can be remedied using the remarkable healing power of lemons, from curing acne and lowering blood pressure to treating varicose veins and rheumatism.

As you read the book and incorporate its principles into your life, never forget that the Lemon Juice Diet is not about getting skinny but about becoming slim. It is a good, healthy

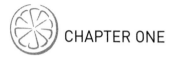 CHAPTER ONE

Lemons: Your Weight-Loss Ally

Before discussing how and why lemons help us to lose weight, it's important to understand the importance of a healthy digestive system.

POOR DIGESTION CAN MAKE YOU FAT

You probably don't need convincing that eating too much and moving too little can make you fat, but what about the part poor digestion plays?

If your digestive system is not working correctly, healthy weight loss becomes almost impossible. Poor digestion can stop your body getting the nutrients it needs to burn fat. It can also interfere with fat burning and cause a build-up of toxins in your body. When toxins build up in your bloodstream, you feel sluggish and depressed; this slows down your metabolism, making your weight-loss goals unattainable.

When your body isn't absorbing the right nutrients – even if you have weight to lose – it is actually in a malnourished state. This means that your brain is constantly craving nutrients and telling you that you are hungry, no matter how many calories you have already consumed or how overweight you are. You may find this hard to believe but large numbers of overweight people with poor digestion are actually starving because their bodies just aren't getting the nutrients they need for optimum health and wellbeing.

It might help to think about weight loss as a race; your goal is to lose weight and boost your health and energy levels. You can see the finishing line in the distance but, with poor digestion, you don't stand a chance of getting there. You are running on a steep incline on a treadmill and going nowhere.

How to Tell if You Have Poor Digestion

Millions of people probably suffer from poor digestion. Many of them have no idea that this is the real reason why they can't lose weight, despite the number of diets they have been on and the hours they have spent exercising. Poor digestion can also be misdiagnosed as depression, IBS (irritable bowel syndrome) and chronic fatigue.

Take a look at the following symptoms. If you suffer from one or more, you may well have a sluggish digestive system:

- Losing weight seems impossible, no matter how hard you try.
- You have been on countless diets and can't really see the point of them any more because they never work.
- You get tired easily, often running out of energy in the early afternoon or in some cases mid-morning.
- You often feel moody, depressed or down in the dumps for no apparent reason.
- Your skin looks dull or you have problems with acne.
- You regularly have indigestion or foul-smelling gas.
- Your bowel movements are inconsistent (constipation or diarrhea are common).

The good news is there is something you can do. Studies have shown that when you restore your digestive system to proper working order you can:

- get the nutrients you need from smaller amounts of food, which causes you to feel less hungry and therefore eat less
- boost your energy levels
- feel healthier and happier
- improve your hair, skin and nails by providing your body with the nutrients it needs
- increase your metabolism
- have normal, regular bowel movements
- lose weight and keep it off

As you can see, you aren't just what you eat; you are also what you absorb from what you eat. The health of your digestive system determines how well nutrients get absorbed from your food, how effectively toxins are filtered out and eliminated from your body, and how quickly you lose weight. This is because the correct nutrients are essential for metabolism and healthy weight loss.

THE DIGESTION-BOOSTING POWER OF LEMON JUICE

Lemon juice is such a great weight-loss ally because it stimulates the flow of saliva and gastric juice and is therefore an excellent digestive agent. When drunk first thing in the morning it also acts as a tonic for the liver, stimulating it to produce bile so that it is ready to digest the day's foods. The beneficial effect lemon juice has on liver function is important because healthy liver function is the key to good digestion.

Some of the most important functions of your liver include:

- metabolising nutrients: breaking them down so that they can be used by the body
- turning toxins into nontoxic substances for expulsion
- manufacturing and excreting bile in order to absorb fat-soluble nutrients and eliminate toxins
- controlling fat metabolism

◯ purifying the blood by filtering bacteria, toxins, antibodies, and other particles from the circulation
◯ manufacturing blood-clotting agents and blood protein

Your overall health and vitality depend greatly on the health of your liver. It's not just important for digestion and detoxification, but also for weight loss. Drugs, alcohol, fatty foods and environmental toxins can overload your liver. When it is overworked it will force the body's other detoxifying agents (your kidneys, adrenals, skin and lymphatic system) to work overtime. This can cause rashes, acne, bloating, yeast imbalances, PMS, constipation and – yes, you guessed it – weight gain. Studies show that liver functions are often disturbed in many overweight people because fat metabolism is so inextricably associated with the liver.

As well as having a beneficial effect on liver function, lemon juice is an excellent digestive aid because of its high citric acid content. Citric acid is found in many fruits and vegetables but its concentration is highest in lemons and limes. The acid content of a lemon can be around 7 to 8 percent – hence its sharp taste. The acid not only protects the fruit from spoiling, but in human metabolism it also combines in a complex interaction with other acids and enzymes to ensure healthy and problem-free digestion by stimulating stomach juices.

Citric acid is relatively mild, in contrast to acids such as sulphuric or hydrochloric acid, and is not powerful enough to break down nutrients on its own. However, as soon as it is in your mouth it gets to work by stimulating your salivary glands. An adequate amount of saliva is important because digestion actually begins in your mouth with your saliva breaking down food as you chew it. Once lemon acid reaches the stomach, either in lemon flesh or as juice, it then supports the first step of digestion in the stomach by stimulating the production of digestive enzymes, such as pepsin, which break down the protein components in food. That's why sprinkling lemon on proteins, such as lean meat, poultry, fish, beans and eggs, will always help you digest them more effectively. Indirectly, therefore, lemon acid supports and promotes the activity of the stomach, preparing the ground for problem-free digestion. In addition, research has shown that it can be highly beneficial in the treatment of a number of digestive problems, such as dyspepsia, constipation and biliousness, and can also destroy intestinal worms and eliminate the gases formed in the digestive tract.

Thanks to its acidity, even a little lemon juice can improve your digestion and lower the impact of any meal on your blood sugar. As you'll see in principle three of the Lemon Juice Diet in Chapter 4, balanced blood sugar levels are extremely important for successful weight loss.

OTHER BENEFITS OF LEMON JUICE

The health and weight-loss benefits of lemons don't just stop at boosting liver function and digestion. Your weight-loss ally has got plenty of other trump cards up its sleeve, including pectin, vitamin C, calcium, quercetin and limonene.

Pectin Power

The lemon is one of the most pectin-rich of all fruits. The tissue of lemon peel alone is comprised of approximately 30 percent pectin. A great source of fiber, pectin can help you lose and maintain your weight because it turns into a sticky gel when you digest it, keeping your stomach from absorbing sugar too quickly. As a result, after eating pectin you feel satisfied for longer. This means that you will eat less, which leads to weight loss. According to a study published in the *Journal of the American College of Nutrition*, pectin eliminates the urge to eat for up to four hours. Pectin can also help to cut cholesterol and blood sugar levels. It may even aid in the prevention of colon cancer.

Vitamin C

Lemon juice is one of the richest and most concentrated food sources of vitamin C, yielding over 90 percent of the vitamin C content of the entire fruit. The juice of just two and a half to three lemons provides the average daily requirement of this vitamin for adults (the RDA for vitamin C is 60 mg a day).

Recent research suggests that people who eat more fresh citrus fruits, such as lemons, limes and oranges, and other fruit and vegetables high in vitamin C are more likely to lose weight. It's not that vitamin C is a new weight-loss wonder drug; what's new is the discovery that consuming an inadequate amount of this vitamin can hinder weight loss. According to researchers from Arizona State University, individuals consuming sufficient amounts of vitamin C oxidize (burn) 30 percent more fat during moderate exercise than those who consume insufficient amounts. In addition, too little vitamin C in the bloodstream has been shown to correlate with increased body fat and waist measurements.

Quercetin

Lemon juice contains high levels of bioflavonoids, particularly quercetin. Bioflavonoids are plant compounds that give plants their color and are found mostly in fruit, vegetables and certain tree barks. They are powerful antioxidants which help protect our bodies from harmful free radicals. They also have antiviral, anticancer and antiallergenic actions. Quercetin is a powerful immune booster that stimulates the production of insulin and helps balance blood sugar levels, freeing the digestive system to process food more efficiently. The result: fewer nutrients are stored as fat. And there's an added bonus to lemon's ability to help balance blood sugar. Swings in blood sugar can prompt hunger pangs, but if blood sugar is balanced hunger fades and less food is consumed.

Calcium Control

As well as being a good source of body-building calcium, lemon juice plays an important role in helping the body to absorb this mineral. Not only does this help prevent osteoporosis but it can also help you lose weight. Research shows that this is because calcium stored in fat cells plays a big part in regulating how fat is stored and broken down in your body. Experts believe that the more calcium there is in a fat cell, the more fat it will burn. So if you want to lose weight you need to make sure you are getting enough calcium, and lemon juice is an excellent alternative to high-fat dairy products.

Limonene

Lemon peel has thousands of tiny glands that produce its essential oil *(Citri aetheroleum)*. This oil contains large amounts of citral, the substance that creates the typical lemony scent and taste, and is also loaded with d-limonene, which studies have shown to protect against a variety of cancers. You don't have to consume much citrus peel to help protect yourself against cancer. As little as one tablespoon of zest per week is enough to make a significant difference. This is equivalent to the peel of approximately one lemon, depending on the size of the fruit and how finely or coarsely the zest is grated.

Research on the Mediterranean diet – one that usually includes parts of the whole lemon and the use of citrus oils – has also shown that citrus peel is beneficial to health and weight loss. Furthermore, those Mediterranean-dwelling people who consume large amounts of citrus fruit have a lower incidence of obesity, cancer and cardiovascular diseases than Europeans living in other areas. A common beverage of the region is lemonade prepared from the whole fruit, including the peel, which adds d-limonene to the diet.

The various parts of a lemon have different proportions of health-boosting substances. According to studies, the main differences between citrus peel and pulp are that the peel contains higher concentrations of d-limonene, as well as other active components known to fight cancer – such as hesperidin, naringin and auraptene – than do the juice and pulp. Gourmet chefs have been using lemon zest for years to add intense, delicious flavor to recipes, and hopefully this book will encourage you to do the same by adding more lemon zest to everyday meals such as soups and salads, or sprinkling it on top of chicken or fish.

This isn't the whole story for lemons; they have many other health-boosting properties. You can find out more about the amazing healing properties of lemons in Chapter 9.

HOW TO LOSE WEIGHT

The way to lose weight and keep it off for good is to get all the nutrients you need from a variety of foods, to eliminate toxins and to keep your liver function and digestion healthy. As we've seen in this chapter, lemon is packed with nutrients that boost digestion and weight loss. Small wonder it's the juice of choice for body-conscious Hollywood stars. So, even if the only change you make after reading this book is to drink a glass of fresh lemon diluted with water every morning or to add lemon peel to your drinks and recipes, you'll still be doing something very positive for your digestion, your waistline and your general health.

It's time to start working with your new weight-loss ally by incorporating lemons and lemon juice into your diet.

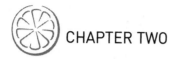

CHAPTER TWO

Your Lemon Juice Diet 24-hour Mini 'Detox'

A body and mind starved of nutrients and overloaded with toxins is one of the major causes of poor digestion, blood sugar swings and the resulting fatigue, mood swings and weight gain. The 24-hour 'detox' in this chapter concentrates on foods and techniques that can help boost your nutrient intake and cleanse your body of toxins naturally.

To ensure your 'detox' is nutritionally sound, the plan will involve drinking plenty of lemon juice with water; it will also involve regular snacks of fruit, vegetables, legumes, nuts and seeds. Rather than starving you of nutrients, which would just cause your blood sugar levels and your mood to sink really low, you will be eating plenty of cleansing, natural foods and drinking lots of water to support your body's own in-house detox system, which is so effective that even the most sophisticated detox product can't compete with it. You'll also learn how to breathe deeply and relax, as research shows that stress can significantly affect your digestion and trigger weight gain, especially around the middle.

The 24-hour plan is a great way to get back on track if you've fallen off the wagon or to give your digestion a boost and kick-start if you're new to all this. As you follow the plan, never forget that healthy eating to lose weight has nothing to do with dieting – we know that diets don't work in the long term – but everything to do with giving your body the best nutrition it can get. So, for the next 24 hours, and hopefully for the rest of your life, you are going to give yourself the very best, top-quality, premium-grade fuel. The basis for this 'detox' diet is four glasses of 'fresh' lemonade, lots of water and regular meals and snacks that are as fresh, natural and healthy as possible. Not only will it give you all the nutrients you need to expel toxins naturally and revitalize your digestive system without feeling hungry, you can also lose a minimum of 1 to 2 pounds, depending on your height and body weight.

Making Your Lemonade

To make your lemonade you will need:

2 tbsp freshly squeezed lemon juice (approximately
   ½ to 1 lemon)
1¼ cups (10 fl oz) pure, filtered water (according to taste)
1 tsp organic grade B maple syrup (optional) or a
   cinnamon stick
Small pinch of cayenne pepper

Mix together the lemon juice, water, maple syrup and cayenne pepper. Stir well and serve at room temperature. As an alternative to maple syrup you could stir a cinnamon stick into your lemon juice. Research has shown that cinnamon can help balance blood sugar and, if you like the taste, it's a fantastic way to add some sweetness.

Use only fresh lemons, organic and vine ripened whenever possible. Never use canned or frozen lemon juice. Mix your lemonade just before drinking. You can, however, squeeze your lemons in the morning and measure out the 2 tablespoons when needed.

The pinch of cayenne pepper adds a zing to the flavor, as well as some stimulating warmth, which speeds cleansing and elimination. Some studies show that the capsaicin in cayenne pepper may increase the body's production of heat for a short time. It may also help to regulate blood sugar levels by affecting the breakdown of carbohydrates after a meal. Based on these studies, capsaicin is being investigated to see if it can be useful in treating obesity. The grade B maple syrup (grade A is over-processed and refined) adds a sweet taste for those who find the drink too bitter, and a welcome shot of zinc and magnesium to help regulate your appetite and further boost fat metabolism.

YOUR LEMON JUICE DIET DETOX DAY: STEP BY STEP

On this one day you will take in enough calories to keep your metabolism running efficiently as well as a host of wholesome and healthy nutrients. Moreover, your body will have 24 hours in which to rid itself of the toxins absorbed by overindulgence, or simply through daily life (stress, pollution and processed food products). You should *not* follow this detox diet for more than one day a week as it is not effective as a general everyday diet. It is, however, highly effective as a cleansing pick-me-up to boost your digestion and get you started on the road to weight loss. It's best to do this detox on a Saturday or Sunday or on a day when you aren't working and bound by your normal routine; then you'll have time to relax and take your time cooking, preparing and eating your food.

Throughout the Day

Make sure you drink at least six to eight glasses of filtered water with added lemon peel. You shouldn't feel any hunger pangs. If you do, drink more water or herbal teas, or have a banana with a handful of mixed seeds or a bowl of warm vegetable soup that isn't high in sodium, additives or preservatives (homemade soup is probably your best option).

First Thing

Try to get up around 7:30 in the morning if you can, and on rising, drink your first glass of lemonade. It's probably best to drink it slightly warm, as cold water first thing in the morning is a shock to the system and can create gas and bloating. Wait at least half an hour until you eat breakfast or until you brush your teeth.

Breakfast

5 each of blackberries, blueberries, raspberries,
    strawberries, and cherries
1 apple
1 pear
1 small container (6 oz) organic live yoghurt
Handful of raw almonds

Chop up all the fruit, mix with the yoghurt and sprinkle with almonds.

Mid-morning Snack

Drink your second glass of lemonade. Ten minutes later have a banana, plus a handful of sunflower or pumpkin seeds.

Lunch

As much mixed green bean or lentil salad as you like, dressed with lemon juice, balsamic vinegar and extra virgin olive oil. You can eat any kinds of beans and lentils, including red kidney, haricot, cannellini, butter, black eye and pinto beans and red, green and brown lentils.

Mid-afternoon Snack

Drink your third glass of lemonade, then 10 minutes later have cucumber, radish and celery crudités, or a handful of raw unsalted nuts and dried fruit.

Dinner

Grilled fish with steamed vegetables (make sure you include onions). You can eat any vegetables you like, fresh or frozen, such as carrots, turnip, rutabaga, Brussels sprouts, cabbage, peppers, mushrooms, corn, leeks, zucchini, broccoli, cauliflower, tomatoes, cucumber, spring onions. You can also choose any of the following fresh fish: cod, flounder, mackerel, salmon, trout, haddock, tuna, shrimp, Dover sole, red mullet, halibut, lemon sole. Make sure you sprinkle your fish with lemon juice before eating. (If you don't eat fish, substitute with soya beans or tofu and avocado.)

OR

Stir-fry a selection of vegetables such as bok choi, spring onions, mushrooms, bamboo shoots and bean sprouts in a little extra virgin olive oil with garlic, lemon juice, ginger and tofu pieces.

About Two Hours before Bed

Have your glass of lemonade, this time with warm or hot water.

Just before You Go to Bed

Have a relaxing warm bath with aromatherapy oils. If you feel hungry after your bath try nibbling on some celery stalks, as they are loaded with magnesium, which is a calming nutrient.

Try to be in bed before 10 P.M. if you can. A good night's sleep is important for weight loss, because lack of sleep disrupts hormones, triggering metabolic changes that mean you don't process food so well. There may also be a link between lack of sleep and increased appetite, so in the weeks and months ahead aim for quality sleep every night; between six and eight hours a night is considered optimum.

GET THE MOST FROM YOUR 24-HOUR DETOX

As well as the above guidelines, there are a few simple rules to follow if you want to get the most from your 24-hour detox:

Drink Water and Lemonade Only

For 24 hours only, drink no coffee or tea (including green tea), or any soft drink. The *only* liquids that are allowed are the four glasses of lemonade made up according to the guidelines above *and* you can drink as much still water (not from a tap unless filtered) and herbal tea as you like. Water is one of the most efficient and natural detoxifying fluids. Not just today but every day you should be aiming for at least six to eight glasses, more if you are exercising.

Don't Smoke

If you are a smoker, try to stop for the next 24 hours. If you cannot manage this, try to limit cigarettes to as few as possible, and do not inhale but smoke the cigarette as you would a cigar. Quitting smoking without gaining weight is outside the scope of this book, but there is overwhelming evidence that smoking is incompatible with a healthy lifestyle. Weight gain is not inevitable if you give up, but it is important that you seek advice about quitting from your physician.

Start Skin Brushing

Buy a skin brush and use it first thing in the morning or last thing at night. Dry skin brushing can help expel toxins from your body because it activates the lymph nodes, a key area of detoxification. Skin brushing should be done when you are dry, not in the bath or shower. You can have a bath or shower afterwards to further boost your circulation, but not during the process. Start by brushing the soles of your feet, working your way up your legs and then your arms and back. Brush lightly and gently towards the heart in long, sweeping movements. Avoid any broken skin, thread veins or varicose veins.

Exercise

Take exercise in any way you want to (walking may be the best) for at least 45 minutes during the day. Try to break into a sweat if you can. If you don't want to go for a walk or a run, put your favorite music on and dance to it for around 40 minutes or in three 15-minute sessions throughout the day. Don't overdo it; just bear in mind that every time you move, flex, stretch and work your body, you are helping lymph fluid to expel toxins.

Breathe!

The way you breathe can have a huge impact on your health because oxygen is a potent detoxifier. Most of us breathe shallowly, thus depriving our bodies of much-needed oxygen.

Oxygen not only feeds your muscles and cells, it also helps detoxify your organs and glands and is just as important as drinking plenty of water and eating healthy food. Indeed, lack of oxygen can starve your body and your brain. Throughout your 24-hour detox day you should try to incorporate deep breathing into your normal activities, such as when you are sitting, chatting, running errands, walking or relaxing.

Stand up Straight

Holding your shoulders back and standing up straight will make you appear taller, give you a flatter stomach, and help you look up to seven pounds slimmer in an instant because standing tall increases the distance between your hips and your ribs.

Don't Multi-task When You Eat

Don't talk with your mouth full, bolt down your dinner, chew gum or have the television or radio on while you eat. You'll swallow more air that way, which makes your stomach bloat.

How to Breathe Properly

1. Begin by lying flat on your back or standing up straight. You may also sit up straight in a chair, if that is more comfortable.
2. Place your hand on your stomach area.
3. Breathe as you normally would and notice whether your hand and stomach rise and fall, or your chest rises and falls, as you breathe.
4. When you are breathing properly, your chest will stay still while your stomach rises slightly as you breathe in. When you breathe out, your chest will continue to stay still while your stomach lowers slightly.
5. To breathe correctly, begin by slowly breathing in through your nose for a count of five while gently pushing your hand up with your stomach.
6. Hold the breath for a count of five.
7. Slowly exhale through your mouth for a count of five while gently pushing down on your stomach.
8. Repeat this process for a few minutes.
9. If you continue to practice breathing this way, you soon will be doing it naturally throughout the day.

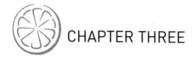 CHAPTER THREE

Getting Started on the Lemon Juice Diet

Before you start incorporating the Lemon Juice Diet principles into your life over the next seven days, here's some useful advice on what foods and drinks to buy and avoid. There are also some guidelines on healthy food preparation and cooking, taking supplements, getting motivated and setting yourself weight-loss goals.

SHOPPING GUIDELINES

A diet rich in fresh, unprocessed foods is the key to good digestion and weight loss, but supermarkets can be daunting places. If you aren't sure exactly what you should be buying to maximize good health and encourage weight loss, the following list can help you decide.

The reasons why you should buy or avoid the foods listed here will become clear in the following chapters, but for now just use it as your at-a-glance shopping guide. Photocopy it and take it with you when you go shopping. If you can, choose organic food. Going organic is a positive step because these foods contain fewer of the chemicals, additives, and other unwanted toxins that have a damaging effect on digestion, deplete the body of nutrients, unsettle hormones and contribute to weight gain and poor health in general. (Visit www.whyorganic.org for more information.)

BEANS/LEGUMES

Beans are an amazing source of nutrients but their nutritional value can be depleted if they are canned or cooked in fat and salt. Avoid frozen beans and beans canned with salt, sugar, and preservatives. Choose instead dried beans or beans canned in water and cooked without animal fat or salt. Most dried beans (not lentils) need to be soaked overnight before cooking. Alternatively, most supermarkets stock canned organic beans that have a little salt added but no unnecessary sugar. Hummus, made from chickpeas, can be bought ready-made from most supermarkets.

BEVERAGES

Avoid alcoholic drinks, coffee, cocoa, pasteurized and/or sweetened fruit juices and carbonated drinks. Choose instead green tea, herbal teas, fresh (preferably organic) vegetable and fruit juices, cereal grain beverages (coffee substitutes), and mineral or filtered water. Black tea (without milk) is fine to drink in moderation, but stick to no more than two to three cups per day.

DAIRY PRODUCTS

These are a source of protein, but avoid soft cheeses, ice cream and artificially colored cheese products as they are high in saturated fat, dyes and preservatives. It is best to avoid low-fat dairy options because they tend to be higher in sugar and make it hard to digest protein and lactose, increasing the risk of poor digestion and nutritional deficiencies. Full-fat products are fine in moderation but try to eat more organic live yoghurt than cheese or milk. Avoid flavored, processed yoghurts and buy organic live yoghurt with the *Lactobacillus acidophilus* culture and add your own fruit instead. Opt for moderate amounts of organic butter or unhydrogenated margarine instead of low-fat spreads, to avoid trans-fatty acids. If you have a milk allergy or intolerance try goat's milk, buttermilk, rice milk, soya milk and all soya products. If you are worried about your calcium intake there are many other foods that contain high levels of calcium, including sesame seeds, leafy green vegetables and nuts.

EGGS

Buy organic, free-range eggs if possible. These won't contain the toxic hormones and antibiotics pumped into factory-produced eggs.

FISH
Avoid all fried fish, shellfish, salted fish, anchovies, herring and fish canned in salt and oil. Choose instead freshwater white fish, salmon, boiled or baked fish and water-packed tuna. Fresh is best but frozen is fine. Freshwater and oily fish are rich in the good fats, known as omega 3, that are essential for reducing cholesterol and promoting health and well-being. They are also low in salt, saturated fat and nutrient-depleting additives.

FRUIT
Fruits are high in essential fiber, vitamins, minerals and antioxidants, but if you aren't buying organic make sure you wash or peel thoroughly before eating to avoid pesticides. Avoid canned and bottled fruit with sweeteners added. Choose instead all fresh, stewed, frozen or dried fruit without sweeteners or the preserving agent sulphur dioxide.

GRAINS
Avoid all white flour products, white rice, pasta, crackers, cold cereals, instant oatmeal and other hot cereals. Choose instead all whole grains and products containing whole grains: cereals, breads, muffins, whole-grain crackers, cream of wheat or rye cereal, buckwheat, millet, oats, brown rice and wild rice. Whole grains are bursting with energy-boosting nutrients and digestion-boosting fiber, unlike refined products which have been stripped of both.

MEATS
Avoid beef, all forms of pork, hot dogs, luncheon meats, smoked, pickled and processed meats, corned beef, duck, goose, spare ribs and organ meats. It's best to avoid meat, especially red meat which has been linked to breast and bowel cancer, but if you want to eat it choose the leaner varieties and go for organic non-breaded, skinless turkey and chicken instead of red meat.

NUTS
Go for all fresh, raw nuts and seeds instead of salted or roasted nuts.

OILS
Choose cold-pressed oils: extra virgin olive oil, corn, safflower, sesame, flaxseed, soya, sunflower and rapeseed oils; margarine made from these oils, and egg-free mayonnaise.

MICROWAVABLE MEALS
Avoid completely.

SEASONINGS
Choose garlic, onions, cayenne, herbs, dried vegetables, lemon juice, seaweed, dulse and pure apple cider vinegar.

SOUP
Avoid canned soups made with salt, preservatives, MSG or fat stock and all creamed soups. Choose instead homemade

soups free from salt, added fats and preservatives, such as bean, lentil, pea, vegetable, tomato, carrot and spinach.

SUGAR
Avoid white, brown or raw cane sugar, corn syrups, chocolate, sweets, fructose, all syrups (except pure maple), all sugar substitutes, jams and jellies made with sugar. Choose instead barley or rice syrup, raw honey, pure maple syrup, un-sulphured blackstrap molasses and Xylitol.

VEGETABLES
Avoid all canned or frozen with salt or additives. Additives added to canned vegetables can deplete essential nutrients called phytochemicals – substances that have incredible benefits for your heart, skin, hair and waistline. Choose instead raw, fresh or frozen vegetables without salt or additives, preferably organic.

COOKING GUIDELINES

Good nutrition to ensure healthy digestion and fat burning is not just a matter of selecting the 'right' foods to eat. It is also important to prepare these foods in ways that will maintain their nutritional benefits. The cooking strategies and recipe substitutes listed below can help retain and, in some cases, improve the nutritional and digestion-boosting value of your favorite dishes. They can also help you meet government recommendations for lower obesity, heart disease and cancer risk, giving you better overall health.

EAT MORE RAW FOODS

The cooking process can destroy valuable nutrients and digestive enzymes. (Eating very hot food isn't good news either because it can trigger stomach upsets as well as gum and throat problems.) This doesn't mean you should go on a diet consisting solely of raw foods as some foods, such as beans, eggs and lean meat, can't be safely eaten until they are cooked. What you need to do is eat more raw food, and whenever you eat a cooked meal make sure you balance it with raw food. It is the combination of raw and cooked foods that works best for your digestion.

PREPARE FOOD CAREFULLY

When cooking fresh foods, your aim should always be to retain as many nutrients as possible. Once fresh food is cut, peeled or opened, the destructive effects of air, light and heat reduce the nutrients in the food by oxidation – even chopping releases an enzyme that kills vitamin C. To avoid nutrient loss, chop vegetables, fruit, nuts, seeds and herbs as near to cooking or serving time as possible. Scrub rather than peel carrots, parsnips and potatoes as many of the health-giving nutrients lie just under the skin. Dress cut vegetables and fruit in lemon juice to minimize nutrient loss. Don't soak prepared vegetable produce as water-soluble nutrients will leach away. A food processor might be a good investment as it makes it easier to chop fresh ingredients just before cooking.

COOK LIGHTLY

Choose cooking methods that will retain flavor, color and nutrients, such as roasting, poaching, steaming or stir-frying. Steam vegetables rather than boiling them, and avoid cooking at high temperatures (except for quick stir-frying) and long cooking times. Extended exposure to heat and liquid can destroy or leach out valuable nutrients, so cook lightly as much as possible. Avoid open-flame grilling of meats as this produces cancer-promoting compounds, and try not to eat charred food.

Fried or heavily grilled foods can produce free radicals and increase your intake of unhealthy fats. If you must fry, add a small amount of water to cold-pressed oil and never let the oil get so hot that it smokes. Stir-frying vegetables is always a healthy cooking method as ingredients are cut into small, thin pieces so they cook very quickly. Nutrients are preserved and very little oil is needed to cook the food.

It isn't yet known whether there are any toxic effects of microwaving food, so it's best to limit it or use only in emergencies.

USE SALT SUBSTITUTES

Instead of adding salt to your food, use herbs, spices, vinegar or lemon juice. There's far too much hidden salt in our diet, and this can cause fluid retention and bloating as well as raising blood pressure. Squeeze fresh lemon juice on vegetables, pasta, soups, rice, fish and stews. It will add so much flavor you'll be able to cut back on salt.

ADD VEG

Add vegetables whenever you can to ensure you get your five-a-day servings. Experiment with more vegetable variety in salads; try new vegetable mixes; include some shredded vegetables in casseroles and add different vegetables to soups and stews. Use lemon peel or chopped red or yellow peppers to 'pep' up the flavor. Try vegetable salsas and fruit chutneys as accompaniments to fish or poultry in place of heavy gravies or sauces.

WATCH THE FAT

Select extra virgin olive oil or sunflower oil. Drain off visible fat while cooking, blot pan-fried foods on paper towels to absorb extra grease, and allow soups to chill before reheating and serving so that the fat can be skimmed off the top.

Reduce the fat in home-baked goodies by substituting up to half of the shortening with stewed apple, puréed prunes, lemon juice and mashed bananas, or yoghurt. It works! Substitute some whole-grain products for white flour in your cooking. Try whole-wheat flour, oatmeal or flax in bread and muffins, or try using some soya flour in biscuits and breads.

OPT FOR LIGHT DESSERTS

Try more fruit-based desserts, such as fresh fruit, stewed fruit and pies, instead of cakes and biscuits. Choose sorbet instead of ice cream. Serve cake with fruit sauce instead of frosting or whipped cream.

CHOOSE GOOD COOKWARE
Stainless steel, cast iron, enamel or glass cookware is best for health. Avoid all aluminum cookware, as this is a heavy toxic metal that can enter food through the cooking process. The same applies to wrapping food in aluminum foil.

Using healthy cooking methods and adding more raw food, vegetables, fruit and whole grains to recipes will help you set a better nutritional table and improve your digestion and health in general.

TAKING SUPPLEMENTS

Nutritional supplements can improve your digestive health because, as you've seen, healthy digestion depends on a range of nutrients that are often lacking in our diet. There is a huge range of digestive supplements available; the ones nutritionists are most likely to recommend are described below.

Vitamin and Minerals
In an ideal world you should be getting all the nutrients you need from your food. However, much of the food we eat today is stripped of essential nutrients due to the manufacturing process and the use of additives, preservatives and pesticides. A good-quality vitamin and mineral supplement is a useful insurance policy, and it's almost impossible to

overdose on nutrients if you take a supplement which contains the RDA (recommended daily allowance). Make sure that your supplement contains the RDA of vitamins A, B, C, D and E plus manganese, chromium, selenium and zinc. These nutrients are all important for digestion and will help support digestion and healthy liver function.

Probiotics

There are trillions of bacteria in your digestive tract and not all of them are good for you. However, if you have enough of the healthy bacteria, they can be your first line of defense against unhealthy bacteria and other viruses that inhibit digestion. The healthy bacteria are known as probiotics and the three main ones are *Bifidobacteria*, *Lactobacillus acidophilus* and *Lactobacillus salivarius*. All these bacteria have been shown to reduce levels of unhealthy bacteria, repair intestinal lining and inhibit disease-promoting microbes.

You can buy probiotic supplements in health food stores, supermarkets and drug stores. However, unless you've been suffering from an infection and need to give your digestive tract a boost, or have been diagnosed a course of probiotics by a nutritionist, there's really no need to take a probiotic supplement every day. It's better for you to get your probiotic fix from fermented food sources such as miso, sourdough bread and sauerkraut, and try to make sure that you have a 'live' natural yoghurt containing *Lactobacillus acidophilus* every day. Including such foods in your diet is a good way to promote healthy intestinal bacteria.

The best food to feed intestinal bacteria is something called fructo-oligosaccharides (FOS), sometimes known as a prebiotic. Bananas, barley, fruit, onions and soya beans are especially rich in these. In general, eating a diet high in fruit and vegetables will promote the growth of healthy bacteria, whereas a diet containing lots of meat is more likely to encourage toxic bacteria.

GOOD ADVICE BEFORE YOU GET GOING

In the early stages of the Lemon Juice Diet, there will be days when you find it hard to stay motivated. Use the following tips to help you back away from the chocolate cake.

Keep a Food Diary
Start writing down everything you eat and drink so that you can check your progress and not allow unhealthy, calorie-rich snacks to creep in. You should also write down your promise to yourself that you are going to eat healthily, lose weight and feel better, and review it when you feel low. This may sound silly, but it really can help you stay on track.

Think Positive
If you feel like giving up because you're down in the dumps, think about how good it is going to feel when you hit your weight-loss target. You need to know what you want from

your weight loss and keep focusing on that. Alternatively, you could conjure up powerful images in your mind of how you will look and feel if things don't change weight-wise.

Find a Weight-loss Partner

If you can't summon up the enthusiasm to exercise or to cook a healthy meal, it can help to find yourself a weight-loss partner. Research shows that people who pair up with a friend to lose weight tend to be more motivated than those who diet alone. Pick your friend carefully though – you need someone who is going to inspire you to keep going, not someone who will encourage you to cheat or who is competitive and makes you feel like a failure. And get your partner and kids to join in too. The Lemon Juice Diet is packed with nutrients that are good for the whole family.

Keep it Interesting

If you are feeling bored with your diet, you're probably eating too much of the same thing. To get slim and fit you need to ditch the idea that healthy food is all about wilted lettuce and tasteless cucumber, and see it as a challenge to get more creative. Promise to try one new fresh food every week. Add flavor with spices and herbs, and up your vegetable quota by making them into main meals instead of just side dishes.

Get Active

If you feel too tired to exercise, you're not alone. A recent survey found that almost 60 percent of people feel they don't have the energy to exercise but the fact is the more you exercise the more energy you have. When you feel too tired to do anything, try acting as if you have loads of energy. Just pretend you are an athlete or a celebrity. This sounds crazy, but if you think about what people with energy would do, this can encourage you to do the same – by so doing, you'll become the kind of person you are modelling yourself on.

Reward Yourself

Celebrate and reward yourself for any success, however small. Treats keep you motivated and boost your self-esteem. But don't celebrate losing 7 pounds by going out for a calorie-laden meal. Go for a massage or to the movies or buy yourself some new clothes instead.

SETTING YOURSELF WEIGHT-LOSS GOALS

You can use bathroom scales or calculations, such as your body mass index (BMI) or your waist-hip ratio, to set yourself weight-loss goals but bear in mind that these calculations offer guesstimates. There are a number of factors that affect your weight, such as fluid retention, hormonal fluctuations and muscle mass, so it's best to take the results you get with a pinch of salt. For example, BMI is affected by how much muscle you have: if you have more muscle, your weight might actually be higher than what is considered healthy on the BMI chart, even though you have a healthy body fat percentage. You need to find what works best for you but the best way to lose weight is to focus less on calculations, numbers and sizes and more on making healthy food choices every day to boost your digestion and fat burning.

If you've set yourself tough goals, like losing seven pounds in a week or never eating chocolate again, you need to get realistic. Set yourself a realistic weight-loss and diet goal, so that you feel like you're achieving something rather than failing. Instead of saying 'I'm going to drop two dress sizes in a month,' aim to tone up your arms and thighs instead. It's a much more specific goal and, by taking the pressure off, you'll find the weight just melts off naturally. Start by introducing just one principle of the Lemon Juice Diet into your life rather than going cold turkey on your junk food vices – soon you'll be introducing two or three more principles and then the remaining three.

Research has shown that gradual weight loss leads to more sustained weight loss. You will lose weight on the Lemon Juice Diet but to make sure it stays off for good you need to do it gradually and set yourself realistic goals.

So when you're considering what to expect from your new eating and exercise plan, be realistic. Healthy weight loss occurs steadily. Aim to lose no more than one to two pounds a week. Losing weight more rapidly means losing water weight or muscle tissue rather than fat. Make your goals realistically achievable 'process goals,' such as eating more fruit and vegetables, rather than 'outcome goals,' such as losing 50 pounds. Changing your process – your habits – is the key to weight loss.

Often, dieters set up 'no-win' situations for themselves by having unrealistic goals and expectations about how 'perfect' they should be and how much weight they should lose. Despite what many of us like to think, nobody's perfect. So every time you vow never to munch your way through a bag of potato chips again or promise that you'll always control your eating, you're setting yourself up to fail by insisting on perfection. To make matters worse, if you violate your own rigid standards, you will be disappointed in yourself and may eat even more because you feel so frustrated.

Remember that to err is human – everyone has setbacks. So, strike imperatives from your vocabulary and aim to eat and live healthily 80 percent of the time. You simply can't eat healthily all of the time, and the occasional treat – a bar of chocolate, an ice cream cone, a double mocha with whipped cream, or a French pastry – doesn't mean you have failed. It's the excesses that are dangerous. It really is important for you to enjoy your food and to allow yourself the odd indulgence. So, although certain foods should be avoided on the Lemon Juice Diet, no food is totally off limits.

(For more tips on making the Lemon Juice Diet a success and staying motivated, especially when you hit a weight-loss plateau, refer to Chapter 8: Staying Motivated.)

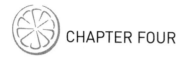 CHAPTER FOUR

The Seven Principles of the Lemon Juice Diet

There aren't any gimmicks or tricks here and you won't be asked to count calories. Remember, the Lemon Juice Diet isn't like other diets. You'll be encouraged to eat *more*, not less, as long as the food you eat is rich in nutrients that can improve your digestion, boost your metabolism and help you lose weight for good.

Below you'll find the seven basic principles of the Lemon Juice Diet, along with the reasons why each principle can help you lose weight and helpful menu suggestions and meal plans. You can follow the meal plans to the letter or use them to get you thinking along the right lines. For recipes and advice on buying, cooking and eating lemons refer to Chapter 6.

You're encouraged to incorporate one new principle into your diet a day over a period of seven days; but by all means give yourself longer if you feel you need it, and don't move on to the next principle until you feel comfortable with the previous one. Sometimes making lots of changes at once can be daunting and overwhelming, so find out what works best for you.

DAY 1

Principle: Drink lemon with water first thing every morning and plenty of water throughout the day.

Make sure you drink a glass of lemon juice and warm water first thing in the morning. You don't need to add the cayenne pepper and maple syrup as you did in the 24-hour mini 'detox' (see Chapter 2). You should also drink more water throughout the day.

Why?

As you saw in the one-day 'detox,' starting your day with a glass of lemon juice and water is a great way to stimulate your digestive system and promote bowel movement. So if you do nothing else, start every single day with a refreshing glass of lemon water! You may want to have one or two glasses later in the day as well. Make sure that you also drink six to eight glasses of water a day, more if you are exercising.

Two-thirds of your body is made up of water. It is impor-tant to keep your liquid intake high as water is essential for all bodily functions. We can exist without food for almost five weeks, but without water we can't last more than a few days.

Water is also crucial if you need to lose weight because it is central to healthy digestion and elimination. It also keeps your skin glowing and your cells working, and it delivers vitamins, minerals and other nutrients to your organs. In addition, for your liver to break down and excrete toxins, you need to drink plenty of water. If you don't drink enough water you will start to feel dizzy, tired and bloated and you could also get stomach upsets.

How?

For your early-morning lemon juice, squeeze one lemon into a glass of warm filtered water. You can use a citrus press to juice the lemon or just squeeze it to get the juice out. Drink it first thing when you wake up, and then go about your normal routine, such as showering and getting dressed. Don't drink or eat anything else for half an hour to give the lemon time to work its magic.

It's really important that you drink between six and eight glasses of filtered water throughout the day, even if you don't feel thirsty. If you are feeling thirsty you could already be dehydrated. Don't drink when you are eating a meal or a snack, though, as this can confuse your digestive system. It's best to do your drinking between meals. By drinking plenty of water between meals you may find that you feel less hungry; sometimes when you feel hungry, you aren't really hungry at all, just thirsty. Remember, too, that if it's hot or you are losing fluids through sweating you need to increase your fluid intake significantly.

Make sure that the water you drink is filtered because much of our tap water is contaminated with nutrient-depleting toxins and chemicals that can unsettle our hormones and create blood sugar imbalances that lead to weight gain. The quickest and easiest way to filter water is to buy a water filter jug, readily available from supermarkets. Use the filtered water for cooking as well as for hot and cold drinks. Alternatively, buy water in glass rather than plastic bottles. A certain amount of residue always dissolves into a drink from the lining of a can or from a plastic bottle, which is why glass bottles are best.

Although pure water is the best drink for quenching thirst and hydrating the body, don't forget that fruit and vegetables consist of 90 percent water.

One way to make sure you drink enough fluids is to fill a jug or bottle with your targeted amount of water and drink it throughout the day. Take it with you in the car or to work, keeping it near you at all times. If the jug is empty by bedtime you know you have achieved your goal.

Although principle number one urges you to drink more, this doesn't include alcohol, tea or coffee. Alcohol is high in calories, so it's best to limit your intake to no more than one small glass a day on the Lemon Juice Diet. Studies show that a small amount of alcohol – particularly red wine – can be good for your heart. It's the same with coffee and tea – you don't need to ban them completely. Studies indicate they can have a beneficial effect on health if less than 300 mg a day is consumed, so make sure you have no more than two or three cups a day. Dieting is not all about deprivation.

Carbonated drinks will just trigger bloating and gas so they're not a wise choice if you suffer from digestive upsets. Water is the best drink for quenching thirst and hydrating your body to prevent fatigue, dry skin, sore eyes and wrinkles – it's even better if you drop in a slice of lemon peel to flavor it. Spritz your water with lemon juice to add flavor (possibly encouraging you to drink more water) and, as you'll see later, to lessen the blood sugar impact of whatever you're eating. Diluted fresh juice is fine but do watch out for fruit juice drinks that pose as fresh fruit juice but are loaded with sugar and additives. There is also a range of good-quality herbal teas available. Finally, it goes without saying that drinking two or three more glasses of lemon juice, in addition to your morning lemon juice drink, is a great way to increase your fluid intake.

Day 1 Meal Plan

Try drinking a glass of water half an hour before each meal and snack to make sure you get your six to eight glasses a day.

First Thing in the Morning

Glass of lemon juice diluted with warm water

Breakfast
Bowl of mixed fruit salad with natural live yoghurt and
	2 tbsp oatmeal
1¼ cups (10 fl oz) glass of soya or organic milk

Mid-morning Snack
8 unsalted almonds
Glass of fresh fruit juice diluted with water

Lunch
Homemade Vegetable Soup (page 112)
2 slices of whole-grain bread filled with salad and a
	sprinkling of grated cheese

Mid-afternoon Snack
2 rice cakes with 1 tbsp cottage cheese and cherry
	tomatoes

Dinner
Grilled fish, tofu or chicken drizzled with lemon and olive
	oil dressing (page 109)
Stir-fried vegetables (selection of leafy greens: kale, bok
	choi and spinach) served with 1 tsp sesame seeds
Baked peaches with cinnamon
Hot citrus comfort drink (page 105)

DAY 2

Principle: Vitamin C power.

Today, as well as drinking your lemon juice first thing and plenty of water throughout the day, you need to eat at least five portions of fruit and vegetables to ensure you are getting enough vitamin C. Ideally, you should aim for two portions of fruit and three to four portions of vegetables. A vegetable portion is approximately 1–1¼ cups of raw vegetables, ⅓–½ cup if cooked. A fruit portion is one medium-sized piece of fruit, such as an apple, banana, orange, or lemon. If you eat the fruit and juice of one raw lemon over the course of the day, plus at least four portions of fruit and vegetables, you will definitely be getting enough vitamin C in your diet.

Why?

All vegetables and most fruits are low-calorie nutritional powerhouses. They are rich in vitamins, minerals, fiber and other nutrients that can boost immunity, balance hormones, calm the nervous system, aid digestion and help you lose weight. One of the most important nutrients for fat metabolism and weight loss, found in abundance in most vegetables and fruit, is vitamin C, of which – as you saw on page 13 – lemons are an optimal source.

Helping control your weight is not the only benefit of eating more fruit and vegetables. Diets rich in fruit and vegetables may reduce the risk of some types of cancer and other chronic diseases.

How?

It may seem hard to fit in so many portions of fruit and vegetables but drinking the juice of one lemon and using the peel in cooking already counts as one. Here are some other really easy ways to get your five-a-day:

- ◯ Chop fruit onto your cereal. It doesn't have to be banana – try pineapple, strawberries or grated apple.
- ◯ Don't forget frozen fruit – it's just as nutritious as the fresh stuff, and is a real convenience food. Try leaving out a bowlful of frozen mixed berries before you go to bed, and then adding yoghurt and a handful of mixed nuts to it in the morning to get a tasty breakfast. Frozen fruit and vegetables are good options when fresh produce is not available. However, be careful to choose those without added sugar, syrup,cream sauces or other ingredients that will add calories.
- ◯ Invest in a juicer and make your own freshly pressed juices such as apple and carrot, banana and apple, apple and celery, mango and pear or whichever fruit you enjoy most.
- ◯ Dried fruit makes a great on-the-move snack as it's easy to carry and packed with fiber. Apricots, raisins, prunes and figs are all tasty options, but be aware that dried fruit can only count as one of your five-a-day, no matter how much of it you eat.
- ◯ Get raw power! Snack on raw veggies such as carrot, celery and cucumber and sprouted vegetables such as alfalfa sprouts. Dip them in salsa and you pack an even greater antioxidant punch.

- Try making or buying vegetable-based soups, such as carrot, tomato or watercress, but if buying avoid salt-laden varieties with additives and preservatives.
- Ensure you always have two types of vegetable with dinner.
- Go for convenience options! These include vegetables that you can throw into the steamer, prechopped mushrooms that you can pan-fry in a couple of minutes, prepared stir-fry mixes and salad leaves.
- Have your finger on the pulse! Beans and other legumes, such as kidney beans, lentils and chickpeas, count toward your total, but only as one portion per day, no matter how much you eat. Add canned mixed beans to a soup, stew or salad.
- Go for as great a variety of color as you can. So, if you're having a green salad, brighten it up with yellow peppers, carrots and tomatoes. This ensures you get the broadest range of health-boosting nutrients.
- Try something new every week. There are bound to be tons of fruit and vegetable varieties that you've never tasted – so vary what you buy and eat.

Day 2 Meal Plan

Whenever you feel hungry today, nibble on fresh vegetables or grab a delicious piece of fruit.

First Thing in the Morning

Glass of lemon juice diluted with warm water

Breakfast
1 poached egg
2 slices of whole-grain toast with a scrape of butter and a
    grilled tomato
1 apple
1¼ cups (10 fl oz) of organic or soya milk

Mid-morning Snack
2 fresh or dried apricots and a handful of unsalted peanuts
Apple, watercress, and lemon juice (page 106)

Lunch
1 tbsp each of red kidney beans, chickpeas and cannellini
    beans mixed with tomatoes, green pepper and lemon
    juice dressing
Whole-grain roll
Large green salad and spring onions
1 kiwi fruit

Mid-afternoon Snack
1 rice cake with cottage cheese and strawberries

Dinner
Vegetable stew (page 127)
Grilled banana with 2 squares of quality dark chocolate
    melted on top

DAY 3

Principle: Balance your blood sugar levels.

After you've drunk your morning glass of lemon juice and made a mental note to get your five-a-day, you can start to think about the next Lemon Juice Diet principle: balancing your blood sugar levels.

Why?

Irritability, mood swings, forgetfulness, anxiety, confusion, poor concentration, weight gain, fatigue and headaches are all symptoms of fluctuating blood sugar levels. Balancing your blood sugar is one of the best ways to trigger weight loss. This is because low blood sugar levels give you powerful cravings – usually for sweet and fattening foods. Also, when blood sugar levels swing too high, so does insulin. This hormone helps shuttle blood sugar (glucose) out of the blood and into your cells to be used as energy. In other words, insulin promotes fat storage – one reason why fluctuating blood sugar levels tend to make you fat. Study after study has shown that high insulin levels are associated with obesity.

How?

When it comes to keeping your blood sugar levels steady, once again lemons are your ally. Sprinkling a couple of teaspoons of undiluted lemon juice over your meals or using the peel and juice in your cooking can lower the impact of that meal on your blood sugar by ensuring that the sugar is released steadily and gradually into your bloodstream. This means that insulin levels don't swing too high and sugar isn't stored as fat. Just one to two teaspoons of lemon juice can be enough to lower the blood sugar impact of a meal by as much as 30 percent. Vinegar can have a similar effect.

Eat Protein

Another great way to keep your blood sugar levels stable is to make sure you eat a little protein with each meal. Protein has a steadying effect on your blood sugar by delaying the absorption of carbohydrates and fats consumed at the same time. It also gives your body an even supply of the amino acids it needs to build and repair cells, and manufacture hormones and brain chemicals. Since your body cannot store protein, you need a constant supply and should eat small portions of good-quality protein with every meal. These include organic whole-grain rice and pasta, whole-grain bread, vegetables, nuts, beans, seeds, soya products, eggs and fish. You will find that incorporating protein into your meals is actually quite simple; for example, for a snack you could have peanut butter on whole-grain toast, rice with beans, or fruit with a handful of nuts and seeds. To help you digest protein better, sprinkle lemon juice over your meal. Serve plenty of lemon slices alongside fish, which wouldn't be the same without them.

Eat Regularly

In addition to using lemon juice, perhaps the best way to keep blood sugar levels stable is to eat regularly. Blood sugar levels and metabolism drop sharply when you go for long periods without meals. Eating five or six times a day will combat food cravings, fatigue and poor concentration, and ensure that your metabolism keeps humming along efficiently, burning fat even when you are resting. The optimum way to plan your meals is to eat a good breakfast followed by a mid-morning snack, a good lunch, a mid-afternoon snack and a light supper. That way you will never get too hungry and your blood sugar levels will remain stable. The aim is to keep your metabolism raised with a regular supply of nutrient-rich foods, so do not go for more than a few hours without a meal or snack.

Eat Breakfast

Remember, it is *never* a good idea to skip meals or fast if you have weight to lose, and you should *always* eat breakfast. Breakfast is, in fact, the most important meal of your day and kick-starts your metabolism – your fat burning – for the day ahead. Studies have shown that people who skip breakfast are often overweight.

Eat the Right Carbs

Another way to keep your blood sugar levels steady is to eat the right carbohydrates. The immediate effect of carbohydrates on your blood sugar is ranked on the glycemic index (GI). Foods low on the GI take longer to convert to glucose, decreasing your risk of weight gain. Brown rice, vegetables and wholemeal breads are typical sources of low-GI carbohydrates. However, refined foods such as sweets, cakes and biscuits, as well as some fruit, tend to raise blood sugar levels too quickly and have a high GI. A quick way to work out the GI of a particular food without resorting to complicated charts is to think about how refined or processed it is. If it is highly refined – that is, it has lots of sugar, salt, additives and preservatives – it is going to send your blood sugar levels rocketing. The less refined it is, the more it will lower your blood sugar.

The GI is helpful if you need to lose weight but it should not be the only tool you use to make food choices. Some high-GI foods, such as carrots, are highly nutritious whereas some low-GI foods, such as a chocolate ice, aren't; and it's pretty obvious which food is better for you. So, if you are thinking about the GI, it's best to consider the GI of your whole meal or snack – that means you can eat higher-GI foods like pineapple, sweet potato and rutabaga to get all their fantastic nutrients if you combine them with a little protein or fiber to slow down the release of sugars. You can also reclaim some of the higher-GI foods such as watermelon and dried fruit by reducing your portion size.

Eat Fiber

Finally, eating plenty of fiber is important for your weight loss because it slows down the release of blood sugar, thus helping to maintain blood–sugar balance. It also keeps your digestion healthy, allowing waste to pass through at a steady rate – this leads to less bloating and fewer toxins being reabsorbed into your bloodstream. Ideally, you should aim to eat around 1–2 oz of fiber daily, and you need to drink plenty of fluid to ensure that it passes through your digestive system. As we saw in Chapter 1, lemons are a fantastic source of fiber, so drinking your lemon juice in the morning, drizzling lemon juice over your meals and using lemon in your cooking will boost your fiber intake. Remember that fruit and vegetables are generally great sources of healthy fiber, as are whole grains, nuts, seeds and legumes. (Don't load up on bran, though, as it's a refined food that won't help your digestion at all.)

Day 3 Meal Plan

Remember: from now on make lemon juice your dressing of choice for salads, fish and meat.

First Thing in the Morning
Glass of lemon juice diluted with warm water

Breakfast
Oatmeal made from 2 tbsp oatmeal and 1¼ cups (10 fl oz) milk with raspberries, strawberries and 1 nectarine

Mid-morning Snack
Fruit salad with lemon dressing
1¼ cups (10 fl oz) of soya or organic milk

Lunch
Warm bean salad (page 122)
Whole-grain roll with scrape of butter
1 small container (6 oz) live natural yoghurt

Mid-afternoon Snack
1 tbsp sunflower seeds
Handful of grapes

Dinner
1 baked salmon steak with lemon juice dressing and large
     selection of steamed vegetables
Small scoop of chocolate ice cream with crushed walnuts

Day 3 Summary

- Eat regular meals and snacks and never skip breakfast.
- Have some good-quality protein with every meal.
- Choose foods that are rich in fiber and as unrefined as possible.
- Sprinkle lemon juice over your meals and use it in your cooking.

There's been a lot to take on board today so you may want to take a few days, or more, to adjust to the recommendations, especially if your diet hasn't been high in fiber, or if you're not used to eating breakfast or drinking less caffeine.

DAY 4

Principle: Cut down on sugar.

We touched on the 'S' word with the last principle: balance your blood sugar levels. But because cutting down on sugar is so important for weight loss, it can be stressed again.

Why?

Although there are many causes and triggers for weight gain, there is one thing on which almost everyone seems to agree: sugar makes it worse. Sugar stimulates the production of too much insulin, causing your blood sugar levels to plummet. If your blood sugar levels aren't stable, not only is the food you eat more likely to be stored as fat but you are also more likely to crave high-calorie, sugar-rich food – which gives you a brief high followed by a big slump. It's a vicious circle which can make weight loss almost impossible and leave you feeling edgy and tired. Sugar can also overwork your liver, disrupting the digestive process by working against good nutrition and depleting your body of nutrients you need to lose weight and feel good. The solution is simple: cut down your sugar intake.

How?

If you feel your blood sugar levels dipping, don't reach for chocolate or sugary foods that can drive them up quickly –

eat something with a lower GI that will give you a steady release of sugar (*see Day 3, page 60*). Bear in mind that refined foods – such as white bread, white rice, instant potato and cornflakes – can act like sugar in your system. It is always best to stick with whole grains and fresh fruit and vegetables, and to eat some protein at the same time.

If you want to monitor your sugar intake, you need to start checking food labels. Sugar is a hidden ingredient in many foods, especially processed ones. It has many different names, including the following: brown sugar, concentrated fruit juice, corn syrup, dextrose, fructose, glucose, honey, lactose, maltose, raw sugar and sucrose. You should get rid of the sugar bowl and opt for fresh rather than canned fruit. Cinnamon, cardamom, nutmeg and other spices can add a sweet flavour without the need to add sugar. Brown and Demerara sugar are sometimes suggested as natural alternatives to white sugar. However, these are virtually the same as white sugar – the only difference is that some of the molasses has been recombined with the refined sugar after processing. These sugars have a glycemic index almost as high as that of white table sugar, so are best avoided.

Finally, if you're wondering why lemon juice hasn't made an appearance yet, that's because the best has been saved to last. Sugar is a very acidic food. Your body thrives on a delicate balance of acid and alkali. Each organ and tissue of the human body has a particular acid–alkali balance (called the 'pH') at which it functions best. The conventional Western diet, rich in sugar and processed foods, affects our pH balance and can leave the body acidic – to the extent that viruses and bacteria are able to take up residence. Your immune system works optimally at an intermediate pH, and can't combat viruses on 'their own turf' at an acidic pH. Certain foods can help us restore balance by taking our pH in a more alkali direction. One of these foods is the lemon. Although lemon juice is itself mildly acidic, it stimulates the production of more acid-neutralizing substances than are needed. When you consume lemon, it neutralizes acid and helps make your body more alkaline, bringing you into better health.

Tips on Cutting Down Sugar

- Don't add it to foods. This is the easiest and most basic way to immediately reduce the amount of sugar you're eating. Your biggest targets: cereal, coffee and tea. If you haven't done so already, throw away the sugar bowl.
- Don't be fooled by 'healthy sugar' disguises. Brown sugar, raw sugar ... it's all pretty much the same thing as far as your body is concerned.
- Make a real effort to reduce or eliminate processed carbohydrates such as white breads, bagels, most pastas and snacks. These are loaded with flour and other ingredients that convert to sugar in the body almost as fast as pure glucose. That sugar gets stored as triglycerides, which is a fancy way of saying fat.
- The natural sugars in fruit can hit your bloodstream fast, so don't eat a piece of fruit without a handful of nuts or seeds to slow down the impact.

- Watch out for 'fat-free' snacks. One of the biggest myths is that if a food is fat-free it doesn't make you fat. Fat-free doesn't mean calorie-free, and most fat-free snacks are loaded with sugar.
- Beware of artificial sweeteners. Unfortunately, they can increase cravings for sugar and carbohydrates.
- Maple syrup is a good substitute for sugar, as long as you don't use too much of it. It is high in trace minerals like zinc and manganese, which are important for fat metabolism.
- Most people digest honey much more easily than sugar. Raw, unpasteurized honey is rich in elements that can help with wound healing, kill bacteria, soothe sore throats and digestive upsets, and decrease local allergy symptoms. Honey is also sweeter than sugar by volume, so you need less in baking or cooking.
- Xylitol is a low-glycemic white crystalline sweetener that occurs naturally in berries, fruit, vegetables, mushrooms and birch trees. In fact, in Finland it is known as 'birch sugar' because the principal raw ingredient in its manufacture is xylan or wood fibre. It is even found naturally in our bodies, and has been shown to be completely non-toxic and safe to take (unlike many other alternative sweeteners).

Detox Warning

If you do decide to cut down on or give up caffeine and to reduce your sugar intake, expect to feel tired or irritable and headachy for a few days. If that happens, drink plenty of water, relax in a warm bath and hang in there; getting over the addiction will do wonders for your appetite, balance and energy.

Day 4 Meal Plan

Whenever you get a craving for something sweet today, go for fresh or dried fruit or a fruit smoothie. (You'll find sweet-tasting fruit smoothie and juice recipes in Chapter 6.) If only chocolate will do, buy a small bar of quality dark chocolate containing at least 70 percent cocoa.

First Thing in the Morning
Glass of lemon juice diluted with warm water

Breakfast
Banana milk shake: blend 1¼ cups (10 fl oz) organic or soya milk, 1 small container (6 oz) of yoghurt, 2 small bananas and 1 tbsp raisins
2 slices of whole-grain toast 1 tsp peanut or almond butter

Mid-morning Snack
Handful of dried fruit and mixed nuts and seeds

Lunch
1 baked potato plus small can of sugar-free baked beans
Large salad with pinch of grated cheese
1 pear or peach

Mid-afternoon Snack
Vegetable sticks with hummus (page 109)

Dinner
Stuffed peppers: mix 4 tbsp cooked basmati rice with 2 tsp
    pine nuts and chopped spring onions, cherry tomatoes
    and 2 oz feta cheese. Cut 1 red pepper in half, remove
    seeds and fill with the rice mixture. Cover with foil,
    bake and serve with large portion of steamed
    vegetables, and lemon poppy seed dressing (page 108).
Baked apple, drizzled with maple syrup and cinnamon

DAY 5

Principle: Forget low-fat.

Your diet should consist of the following:

- 25 percent healthy protein: nuts, seeds, eggs, leafy green vegetables, beans and fish with bones
- 40 to 50 percent healthy carbohydrates: organic whole grains, legumes, vegetables and fruit
- 25 percent healthy fats: nuts, seeds, oily fish, extra virgin olive oil and light vegetable oils

So, far from being something to avoid, fats – in the right form – make up a significant proportion of a healthy diet.

Why?

Lots of us have spent years following low-fat diets. While it's true that fat is high in calories, it's also a fact that you need fat in your diet in order to lose weight. You just need to make sure you are eating the right kinds in moderate amounts.

If your diet is too low in fat you could suffer from mood swings, joint pain, infertility, skin problems and weight gain. Healthy fats can help with weight loss because they delay the passage of carbohydrates into your bloodstream, keeping your blood sugar levels stable and your insulin down.

How?

As a guideline, around 20 to 25 percent of your diet should come in the form of good fats. These include:

- omega 3 and 6 essential fatty acids (EFAs), found in nuts, seeds and oily fish (mackerel, salmon, herrings, sardines and tuna) – excellent hormone regulators and blood sugar stabilizers
- unsaturated fat, found in extra virgin olive oil

You can also increase your intake of linolenic acid, the substance your body uses to manufacture another essential fatty acid – gamma linolenic acid – by including light vegetable oils in your diet, such as sunflower or soya oil. Perhaps the simplest solution is to use flaxseed or hempseed oil, which contains both linolenic and omega 3 acids.

On the other hand, you should avoid:

- saturated fats, found in red meat, cakes and pastries
- trans-fatty acids, found in many commercial foods

These are low in nutrients and rich in substances that can increase your risk of heart disease and obesity.

In a nutshell, aim to eat fish at least twice a week, with one portion being oily fish. Sprinkling lemon juice over your fish will improve not only the flavor but the digestibility of your whole meal too. You should also eat a small handful of nuts and seeds (linseeds, sunflower seeds, pumpkin seeds, hemp seeds, almonds, walnuts) daily as a snack between meals. You can take flaxseed oil daily by the tablespoon or mixed with lemon juice in salad dressings.

Day 5 Meal Plan

If you're not sure whether or not you are getting enough essential fats in your diet you have everything to gain and nothing to lose by taking a fish oil or flaxseed oil supplement.

First Thing in the Morning
Glass of lemon juice diluted with warm water

Breakfast
1 slice of rye bread with 1 sliced hard-boiled egg and
    1 sliced tomato
6 or 7 strawberries

Mid-morning Snack
Handful of nuts
1¼ cups (10 fl oz) of soya milk

Lunch
Open sandwich with cucumber and smoked salmon
    (page 117)
1 small container (6 oz) of live natural yoghurt

Mid-afternoon Snack
1 peach
A handful of grapes
A handful of sunflower seeds

Dinner
Tuna and corn pasta: mix 6 tbsp (3 oz) cooked whole-wheat
    pasta with a small can of tuna in water, 2 tbsp corn,
    and a small jar of tomato sauce. Heat through and
    serve with steamed vegetables and lemon juice
    dressing
Dried fruit compote (page 130)

DAY 6

Principle: Eat lots of fresh whole foods.

'Whole foods' means foods that are unrefined and in their most natural form – vegetables, fruit, whole grains, whole-wheat pasta and rice and legumes, such as peas and beans – which are naturally full of nutrients. Whole foods do not contain any additives such as artificial colorings or preservatives.

Why?

Whole foods are bursting with nutrients your body needs for good health and weight loss. They contain plenty of fiber, which has a stimulating effect on the digestive system and can slow down the conversion of carbohydrates into glucose. Best of all, though, whole foods – especially when organic – are free of hidden sugar and unwanted chemicals that overload your liver, making it hard for your body to digest food efficiently and burn fat. Eating as many fresh whole foods as you can will boost nutritional support to your body's detox system.

There's even more detox power in fresh food when it's raw or as close to its natural state as possible. Raw food is loaded with enzymes that work tirelessly in breaking down food, assisting the digestive system, boosting immune function, carrying on the functions of metabolism and removing toxins from the body.

How?

If you've been following the Lemon Juice Diet guidelines you should already be eating plenty of fresh healthy food and avoiding refined foods that are high in sugar and fat. Lemon is a nutrient-packed whole food, and waking up to a glass of lemon water is a fantastic way to start your day as you mean to go on – with the emphasis on foods and drinks that are as fresh and as healthy as possible.

Choose brown pasta, whole-grain bread and cereals and eat lots of vegetables and fruit. Try to have fresh soups, smoothies and juices (not from concentrates) and eat a side salad with every meal. This isn't to say you should always eat fresh raw food – your digestive system couldn't take that – but it is a good idea to eat more of it and to try to cook less. Here are some easy ways to incorporate more fresh food into your diet:

- Soups and salads made from fresh vegetables, grains and legumes are easy to prepare and store.
- Tiered steamers can be used to cook fresh fish and vegetables at the same time. Steaming is the healthiest way to cook your veggies because, unlike boiling, it retains the most nutrients.
- Keep fresh fruit and vegetables handy at all times, even at work.
- Add your own fresh vegetables and toppings to pizza bases.
- Whole-grain bread with chicken, tuna or tofu with a side salad makes for a quick and fresh light meal.

⬭ Always order a side salad when you eat out, but leave the dressing or have it on the side so you can add your own.

Fresh food can become unhealthy food if it is cooked unhealthily, so make sure you follow the cooking tips on page 36 (*Chapter 3*).

A Lighter Evening Meal

Whole foods such as wholegrain bread, pasta, cereal and rice are best eaten during the day rather than as your evening meal. Restricting your carbohydrate intake in the evening will automatically help you reduce your calorie intake without the need to count calories or deprive yourself of the important carbohydrates you can have at breakfast and lunch. It will also help you get more nutrients from fruit and vegetable sources in the evening meal and reduce the risk of bloating.

Know What You Are Getting

To make sure the food you eat is as fresh and as natural as possible, and free of unwanted toxins and chemicals, going organic is your best option. Organic food is produced to more 'natural' standards. Few, if any, chemicals are used and most pesticides are banned or very carefully controlled.

You also need to get into the habit of reading food labels to see just how many additives and preservatives you are overloading your liver with. It's impossible these days to ensure everything you eat is fresh and toxin-free, so if you do need to buy packaged food make sure you go for the one with the shortest list of chemical ingredients. The shopping guidelines in Chapter 3 (*page 31*) will also help you make the right choices.

Day 6 Meal Plan

Remember today to increase your intake of raw fruit and vegetables because if you're eating food raw it's more likely to be fresh and natural.

First Thing in the Morning
Glass of lemon juice diluted with warm water

Breakfast
1 bowl of fresh fruit salad
1 small container (6 oz) of low-fat natural yoghurt and
    2 tbsp rolled oats
1¼ cups (10 fl oz) of organic or soya milk

Mid-morning Snack
1 nectarine
Handful of mixed nuts and seeds

Lunch
1 small avocado mixed with 4 oz of shrimp
Salad dressed with lemon juice, olive oil and balsamic
    vinegar
1 apple

Midafternoon Snack
Slice of whole-grain toast with grated Cheddar cheese and
    1 tsp Marmite or 1 tsp peanut or almond butter

Dinner
Omelette made using cooking spray, sliced mushrooms, 2
    eggs, 3 tbsp grated cheese
Steamed vegetables
1 small banana
Handful of strawberries

DAY 7

Principle: Know your digestion do's and don'ts.

Why?

As we have seen, if your digestion is poor you won't be getting the nutrients you need to boost your metabolism and shift excess weight, however healthy your diet is. If you're drinking a glass of lemon juice water every morning and following the principles of the Lemon Juice Diet, your digestion will have already improved, but to give it that final push, incorporate the following tips into your diet and lifestyle.

How?

Chew it Over

If you don't chew your food properly you give more work to the rest of the digestive system, putting it under stress. As well as making food easier to swallow, saliva contains enzymes that contribute to the chemical process of digestion. If food is not properly chewed, nutrients remain locked in the food and do not help you, and undigested matter feeds bad bacteria; this can lead to bacterial overgrowth, gas, and other symptoms of indigestion. Chewing also relaxes the lower stomach muscle and triggers nerve messages that activate the whole digestive process. Aim to chew food until it is small enough to swallow easily. As a rule of thumb, if you can tell what kind of food you are eating from its texture, not its taste, you haven't chewed it enough.

Eat Properly

Put your knife and fork down between mouthfuls and take your time. How you eat is as important as what you eat for a healthy digestion. Keep your portions moderate, eat at regular times (your digestive system works best when it knows what to expect), and, don't forget, take all the time you need to chew every mouthful and savor every bite.

Don't Sweat the Small Stuff

Your stomach and intestines are very sensitive to stress, and when you feel anxious your digestion shuts down to help your body focus on preparing the fight-and-flight response. This means that food is only partially digested, leading to poor digestion and eventually to nutrient deficiency. If stress is long term, in time the body will gradually become less able to produce stomach acid and digestive enzymes because it is in a constant state of alert. Finding ways to manage and cope with stress is important for your digestive health, as well as your emotional health. The Lemon Juice Diet can play a significant role in helping you cope with stress, as can getting a good night's sleep and finding ways to relax and switch off. (*See also the tips on stress-proofing your life on page 163, Chapter 8.*)

Don't Eat When You Are Tired

Never eat when very tired, mentally or physically. And never eat a meal within two hours of bedtime. A light snack is fine if you are really hungry but remember when you go to bed your body needs to be resting, not digesting.

Turn off the Television

If you eat when watching television, you won't be concentrating on your food and so you are likely to eat way too much. Overeating will make your heart pump harder and your stomach work too hard. The excess food will not be digested properly and therefore not made available to your bloodstream in molecules small enough for proper use by the body and you don't need reminding that excess food tends to end up as excess fat.

Give it 20 Minutes

If you have finished your meal and still feel hungry, wait 20 minutes before eating more. It takes about 20 minutes for your brain to catch up with your stomach and recognize that you are full.

Be Active

Regular aerobic activity (at least 30 minutes of any activity that makes you feel slightly breathless and sweaty, five or six days a week) helps stimulate the muscles of the digestive system, enabling you to digest food better and expel waste more efficiently. A gentle walk, about 20 minutes after a meal, also activates your digestion. (*See Chapter 7 for more tips on how simple exercise can help melt the pounds away.*)

Day 7 Meal Plan

Well done for completing your first week on the Lemon Juice Diet. Celebrate today by giving yourself plenty of time to cook, chew and really enjoy your food.

First Thing in the Morning
Glass of lemon juice diluted with warm water

Breakfast
Whole-grain cereal with fresh fruit and seeds
Organic milk
Glass of diluted fresh apple juice

Mid-morning Snack
½ cup of guacamole with carrot sticks
1¼ cups (10 fl oz) of soya or organic milk

Lunch
Veggie pizza: cut a 4-inch whole-grain pita in half. Top with 4 tbsp tomato sauce, sliced mushrooms and green pepper, 1 tbsp corn and small ball of mozzarella cheese, sliced. Bake until the cheese melts.

Mid-afternoon Snack
Fruit salad with sunflower seeds

Dinner
Risotto (page 115)
Red fruit dessert (page 133)

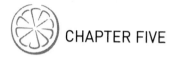 CHAPTER FIVE

Beyond the First Week

The following menu suggestions will help you stay with the Lemon Juice Diet. They will boost your digestion and keep your blood sugar levels balanced so that you lose weight and feel lighter, brighter and full of bounce. Just choose one option from each section every day. Follow these suggestions for the next three to four weeks, then, after your first month on the Lemon Juice Diet, you can use them as a foundation for your own meal plans and recipes.

A few tips and reminders:

- Don't forget to drink plenty of water, herbal teas and diluted fruit juices and cut out as much caffeine, alcohol and carbonated drinks as you can.
- As well as meals and snacks, have an extra 1¼ cups (10 fl oz) of soya or organic milk every day so you don't miss out on bone-strengthening calcium.

- Feel free to eat plenty of fresh raw salad and vegetables, including all leafy greens, spring onions, fresh tomatoes, peppers, bean sprouts, cucumber, herbs and spices.
- It's unlikely, but if you do feel hungry between your meals and snacks, choose an apple plus a couple of dried apricot pieces, a dried fig and some fresh nuts or some celery sticks and vegetable dips.

METABOLISM-BOOSTING BREAKFASTS

Remember: *never* skip breakfast. First thing, have a glass of lemon juice diluted with warm water, then half an hour later try one of the following:

1 scrambled egg, 2 grilled tomatoes and 2 small slices of
whole-grain toast with low-fat spread
Glass of diluted fresh pineapple juice

Slice a banana and add to oatmeal made with soya milk,
chopped prunes, nuts and seeds
1 pear
Glass of diluted fresh apple juice

2 slices of whole-grain toast with 2 tbsp peanut butter
Half a grapefruit

1 scrambled egg and grilled mushrooms on 1 slice of
whole-grain toast

Glass of diluted fresh fruit juice

2 slices of whole-grain toast with butter and Marmite
1 apple
Glass of diluted fresh fruit juice

1 small container (6 oz) of live yoghurt
1 Shredded Wheat or Weetabix
3 oz of fresh berries
Glass of diluted fresh apple or orange juice

Half a pink grapefruit with 1 tsp maple syrup
1 slice of whole-grain bread or toast with scrape of butter
1 medium-sized boiled or poached egg

Fruit smoothie made from mixed berries, soya milk and
    1 tbsp ground or soaked linseeds

Oatmeal made with skimmed milk or soya milk topped
    with 1 tsp honey and 1 tbsp nuts and seeds, such as
    almonds, linseeds and sunflower seeds
Glass of diluted fresh fruit juice

Fruit salad, including pineapple and papaya, sprinkled with
    1 tbsp ground nuts, such as almonds, linseeds and
    sunflower seeds
1¼ cups (10 fl oz) of soya or skimmed milk

Sugar-free baked beans on whole-grain toast
Piece of fresh fruit

1 slice whole-grain toast with cottage cheese, small cup of
blueberries and a handful of toasted almonds
Glass of diluted fresh fruit juice

Oatmeal made with 1¼ cups (10 fl oz) of organic milk or
soya milk with small chopped banana, ½ tsp cinnamon
and some berries
Glass of diluted fresh fruit juice

2 Weetabix or Shredded Wheat with hot milk, raisins and ½
tsp cinnamon
Glass of diluted fresh apple juice

MID-MORNING PICK-ME-UPS

Don't reach for chocolate. Try the following instead:

Freshly squeezed orange, lemon, or grapefruit juice
Small handful of mixed nuts and seeds

Bowl of strawberries and raspberries
1 small container (6 oz) of live natural yoghurt

Strawberries and 1 kiwi fruit
1 small container (6 oz) of live natural yoghurt

Piece of fresh fruit with handful of mixed nuts

Oatmeal with 1 cup skimmed milk topped with 2 tbsp
sultanas

1 tbsp unsalted peanuts
2 dried apricots

1 tbsp almonds and sunflower seeds

1 small square Cheddar cheese
1 rice cake

4 brazil nuts

1 small container (6 oz) of live yoghurt with nuts and seeds

1 slice of whole-grain toast with a scrape of butter or a
little Marmite

1 boiled egg
Salad with lemon juice dressing

1 peach
Handful of grapes and sunflower seeds

Vegetable sticks with hummus (page 109)

Banana and pineapple smoothie (page 107)

Pasta salad (page 128)

Energizing Lunches

Have a small amount of healthy carbohydrates with your lunch, such as whole-grain bread, brown rice or pasta.

Potato and vegetable salad (page 124)

Mexican bean salad (page 123)

1 cooked skinless chicken breast or grilled tofu slices
5 tbsp whole-wheat pasta
Green salad drizzled with lemon juice

Hummus (page 109) with pita and vegetable crudités
1 apple

Vegetable stew (page 127)

Open-face tuna and salad sandwich on whole-grain bread
     with 3 tbsp (1½ oz) avocado
A portion of salad with low-fat lemon juice dressing (made
     with lemon juice, balsamic vinegar, olive oil and garlic
     with herbs and spices of your choice)

Zucchini and ricotta salad (page 126)

Egg and tuna roll made with a 2½ oz whole-grain roll; 1
     boiled egg, ¼ cup (2 oz) tuna and 1 dessert bowl of
     salad leaves drizzled with lemon, served with 3 tbsp
     (1½ oz) chopped avocado

Tomato and basil soup with 1 tbsp grated Parmesan cheese
1 slice of whole-grain bread

Whole-grain pita bread stuffed with tuna or cottage cheese
Piece of fresh fruit

Homemade vegetable soup (page 112)
Whole-grain roll
Cottage cheese

Warm bean salad (page 122)

Large mixed salad including watercress, broccoli, beet, peppers and tomatoes. Toss in olive oil and lemon juice and season and sprinkle with nuts and seeds or add a 6 oz can of tuna in spring water

1 grilled tuna steak and steamed vegetables
1 large boiled potato mashed with 1 tbsp pesto
1 small container (6 oz) of live natural yoghurt

Grilled salmon fillet
6 tbsp (3½ oz) brown rice or 3 new potatoes
Peas and salad
Fruit compote with low-fat natural yoghurt

Homemade tomato, pepper and onion soup with whole-grain roll

1 baked potato
1 small can of low-sugar baked beans
3 tbsp grated reduced-fat cheese
Salad drizzled with lemon juice

Mackerel salad: place a roughly chopped 6 oz fillet of
smoked mackerel and a portion of butter beans on a
large handful of watercress and rocket dressed with
lemon juice

5 oz cooked whole-grain tagliatelle mixed with steamed
broccoli, 4 tbsp corn and 2 tbsp low-fat soft cheese
1 meringue nest filled with berries and 1 tbsp light cream

Lightly grilled tuna steak served with 3½ oz brown rice and
stir-fried mixed vegetables including shredded
cabbage, broccoli, peppers, spring onions and
carrots

Tuna salad with soy nuts (page 121)

Veggie pizza (page 81)
Salad with lemon juice dressing

MID-AFTERNOON REVIVER

Try drinking another glass of lemon juice with water, then about 10 minutes later have a snack to crank up your energy levels and take away any hunger pangs:

Vegetable soup (page 112)

Lentil soup (page 111)

Carrot soup (page 113)

2 rice cake topped with low-fat cottage cheese and cherry tomatoes

1 small (6 oz) can of wild salmon with celery or asparagus

10 raw almonds

Handful of unsalted peanuts
2 dried ready-to-eat apricots

Handful of almonds and pumpkin seeds

1 apple
3 fresh almonds

1 tbsp dried fruit and unsalted nuts

2 handfuls of raw vegetables: dip carrots, celery, pepper, mushrooms or zucchini in 1 tbsp hummus or salsa

2 squares of dark chocolate (at least 70 percent cocoa solids)

Rice cake with mashed avocado to spread

Fresh apple, carrot, ginger or lemon juice
4 whole almonds

Slow-Burn Dinners

Don't slump in front of the television when you get home or after you've eaten dinner; go for a short walk instead. Remember that now isn't the time to be loading your plate full of carbohydrates in the form of bread, pasta, cereal and rice as this will only lead to bloating. So, if you want a flat tummy in the morning, add as much salad and as many raw or steamed vegetables to your meal as you like. Remember to drizzle your salads and fish with lemon juice. And don't be afraid to treat yourself to a scoop of low-fat chocolate ice cream now and again.

Grilled salmon steak served with green or brown lentils and steamed broccoli
Soya yoghurt and a sprinkle of mixed nuts

White fish fillet, cooked with a squeeze of lemon, pinch of
     black pepper and dill
Large portion of salad
Fruit salad made up of your favourite fruit, such as mango,
     banana, berries, apple or lemon – cut into bite-sized
     chunks and toss with some fresh mint leaves

Grilled chicken breast or tofu with fresh pineapple and
     coriander salsa
Stir-fried rice noodles and vegetables, such as broccoli,
     snow peas and baby corn
Frozen summer berries with fat-free natural yoghurt and a
     drizzle of honey

Marinated shrimp, sweetcorn and chickpea salsa
Fruit and nut salad

1¼ cups (4 oz) of large peeled shrimp
Large salad of mixed green leaves, cucumber, spring
     onions, cherry tomatoes and thinly sliced red peppers
     dressed with 1 dsp extra virgin olive oil and a drizzle of
     lemon juice and apple cider vinegar
Grilled fruit

Vegetable stew (page 127)
Dried fruit compote (page 130)

Grilled chicken or marinated tofu kebabs with roasted
     Mediterranean vegetables and hummus
Baked apple with low-fat natural yoghurt

Grilled fish served with lightly steamed asparagus drizzled
with extra virgin olive oil and lemon juice
Large mixed salad
Homemade mixed berry compote with 1 tbsp fat-free
natural yoghurt

Risotto (page 115)
Red fruit dessert (page 133)

Shrimp salad (page 120)
Small slice of lemon almond cake (page 134)

Baked salmon
Large mixed salad with half an avocado sprinkled with nuts
and seeds and dressed with extra virgin olive oil and
lemon juice
Fruit and Ryvita dessert (page 132) with a small scoop of
ice cream

Lemon-crusted salmon (page 118)
Banana surprise (page 131)

Chicken ginger skewers (page 114)
Fruit kebabs with lemon cream (page 130)

Chicken or tofu salad made with 3½ oz cooked chicken or
tofu, large bowl of salad vegetables, ¾ oz avocado, ¾ oz
feta and oil-free lemon juice dressing
Banana surprise (page 131)

Mixed bean salad with tomatoes, half an avocado, walnuts,
cucumber, peppers and olive oil with lemon juice
dressing
Baked apples with stuffing (page 131)

Tuna or salmon fish cakes
Steamed vegetables

Egg and spinach cake (page 129)
Steamed vegetables or large green salad
Fruit kebabs with lemon cream (page 130)

EATING MORE, NOT LESS

The Lemon Juice Diet is all about eating more, not less, as
long as the foods you eat are as natural, unprocessed and
nutritious as lemons. This means cutting down on sugar,
additives, preservatives and salt, but it also means piling
your plate high with foods rich in nutrients.

Forget calorie counting; the way to lose weight and to
keep it off is to boost your nutrient intake so food is digested properly, hormones and blood sugar levels are balanced,
metabolism is fired up and fat burning can begin. As previ-
ously stated, if your body isn't getting the nutrients it needs,
it will cling stubbornly to every ounce of fat because it fears
that starvation might be around the corner. If you've been
following the digestion-boosting Lemon Juice Diet meal
plans in the last few days or weeks, what you've been doing

is reassuring your body – with regular meals and snacks rich in vitamins, minerals and other nutrients – that there is going to be a steady supply of nutrients and that it is perfectly safe for you to lose weight.

It's also safe for you to enjoy your food. As long as you eat healthily at least 80 percent of the time, you can afford the occasional indulgence. Variety is the key to success in healthy eating, weight loss and in life, so make sure you enjoy your Lemon Juice Diet. Remember, it's not just about lemons, but about eating a healthy, satisfying and varied diet so you have all the energy you need to live your life to the max.

NAVIGATING THE LOW POINTS

Just over a week into your Lemon Juice Diet and you should already be feeling more energetic and your clothes should be slightly looser. You'll also notice that bloating, which can make you feel so uncomfortable, is slowly but surely easing. You'll have achieved this without a hint of nutritional deprivation but this isn't to say there won't be low points along the way. Most diets make great claims about weight loss but forget to mention how tough things can be when you change the way you eat.

The fact is that on the Lemon Juice Diet there may be times when you feel out of sorts because your body has stopped eating the foods it is used to. These symptoms are entirely normal and to be expected when you begin a healthy eating plan; the good news is they will pass in a few days. If the going gets really tough there's more motivational advice to keep you on track in Chapter 8: Staying Motivated.

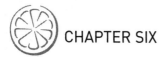 CHAPTER SIX

The Lemon Juice Diet Recipes

To get the greatest benefits from the nutrients in lemons, here is what to look for when you buy them and what you need to know when cooking and eating them.

BUYING, STORING AND JUICING LEMONS

Buying Lemons

Lemons, scientifically known as *Citrus limon*, are the fruit that evokes images of sunshine. While most lemons are tart, acidic and astringent, they are also surprisingly refreshing.

The two main types of sour lemons are the Eureka and the Lisbon. The Eureka generally has more textured skin, a short neck at one end and a few seeds, while the Lisbon has smoother skin, no neck and is generally seedless. In addition to these sour lemons, there are also some varieties that are sweet in flavor. One notable example is the Meyer lemon that is becoming more popular in both markets and restaurants. Although they are available throughout the year, lemons are in their peak season between May and August.

The size of the fruit does not indicate the amount of juice it will give you. Small lemons with a thin peel generally give you more juice than varieties with thick peels and comparatively little flesh.

Ripe lemons are not hard; the skin is shiny and an even, light yellow. If the fruit has green spots and looks matte, it is not ripe. It is overripe if the skin is deep yellow and soft to the touch, or if the skin is wrinkled or torn.

It's best to purchase organic lemons, since lemons can often be sprayed with chemicals and pesticides. If organic isn't possible, soak the whole fruit in lukewarm water with a small amount of dishwashing liquid, then scrub and rinse in cold, clear water.

Storing Lemons

Lemons will keep for around eight to ten days at room temperature. If you want to keep them for longer, preserve their quality by refrigerating them in a container that allows plenty of air around the fruit. Lemons can also be frozen for up to six months. To freeze the juice, pour it into ice-cube trays. Once thawed, the taste and quality is as if it were freshly squeezed. If you cut a lemon in half and want to save the rest for future use, brush the cut side with vinegar to keep the half lemon fresh for a few days.

Pressing Juice

It is best to press lemons for juice at room temperature. The juice is hidden in tiny sacs that need to burst before pressing. To extract the juice, place the lemon on a hard surface and use your palm to roll it backwards and forwards several times before exerting firm pressure. It's probably best to squeeze lemons over a sieve or colander to remove the seeds. Squeezing the lemons by hand, upright over a bowl, really doesn't keep the seeds out of the food. With lemon presses, the sacs are burst through repeated pressure against the ridges of the lemon press. If you only need a little bit of lemon juice, pierce the lemon with a skewer or toothpick and squeeze out the amount you want, then rinse with water and place back in a container in the refrigerator. You will get more juice if you soak the lemon for a few minutes in warm water. With this treatment the average lemon should yield around 2 to 3 tablespoons (1½ fl oz) of juice.

Using the Peel

Lemons can be bought waxed or unwaxed. Choose unwaxed lemons if you're using the zest, adding slices to drinks or using as a garnish. Waxed are fine if you're just using the juice. If you can't buy unwaxed lemons then a good scrub with a vegetable brush will remove most traces of wax. You can tell if lemons are waxed because they look shinier and feel smooth when you rub your thumb along them.

When peeling lemons, you're removing the zest, or colored part of the skin. Use a grater with tiny holes, or a lemon zester, which has small loops of wire to remove the rind, taking care not to remove the white pith with the zest because it is very bitter. Once peeled, the strips should be spread out on waxed paper left to dry for two days, and then kept in a cotton pouch in a dry, airy place. The drying can be speeded up in the oven. Place the strips of peel on a baking sheet and dry them at the lowest heat setting for four hours, leaving the oven door slightly open. Before using the lemon peel, soak it in water until softer.

Once you have removed the peel, make sure you use the lemon as soon as possible. Without the peel lemons spoil and become moldy and harmful very quickly. You can, of course, buy ready-made lemon peel.

Some Quick-Serving Ideas for Lemons

- Place thinly sliced lemons, peel and all, underneath and around fish before cooking. Baking or grilling will soften the slices so that they can be eaten along with the fish.
- Combine lemon juice with olive or flax oil, freshly crushed garlic and pepper to make a light and refreshing salad dressing.
- Serve lemon wedges with meals, as their tartness makes a great salt substitute.
- Add a zing to lunch by tossing seasoned cooked brown rice with garden peas, chicken or tofu pieces, spring onions, pumpkin seeds, lime juice and lemon zest.
- Squeeze some lemon juice on to an avocado quarter and eat as is.

RECIPES

After reading this book, cooking without lemons will be almost unimaginable. In all the low-fat, low-GI, nutrient-packed recipes that follow, you'll find that the unique properties of lemons combine with the other ingredients for optimal health and weight-loss benefits, as well as taste. Use these recipes as a starting point to get you thinking along the right lines and then go on to create your own lemon recipes, using lemons, lemon juice or grated lemon peel for seasoning. Just try to remember one thing: nothing adds zest and fat-fighting power to a dish like a squeeze of lemon.

Note: Unless otherwise stated, recipes serve one.

Drinks and Juices

LEMON MINI 'DETOX' DRINK

2 tbsp freshly squeezed lemon juice (approximately ½ to 1
    lemon)
1¼ cups (10 fl oz) pure, filtered water (according to taste)
1 tsp organic grade B maple syrup (optional) or a
    cinnamon stick
Small pinch of cayenne pepper

Mix together the lemon juice, water, maple syrup and
cayenne pepper. Stir well and serve slightly warm at room
temperature.

LEMONADE

6 lemons
1¾ pints water
2 tbsp maple syrup
Ice cubes
Fresh peppermint leaves

Take the zest of 1 lemon and the juice of all 6, mix with water
and maple syrup. Stir well and chill. Serve with ice cubes
and a few fresh peppermint leaves.

HOT CITRUS COMFORT

2 lemons, juiced
1¼ cups (10 fl oz) hot water or brewed tea of your choice
2 tsp maple syrup
½ tsp ground ginger
½ tsp ground cinnamon

Put the juice in a small saucepan. Stir in the water or tea, syrup, ginger, and cinnamon. Allow to boil, and then simmer for a few minutes before serving.

APPLE, PEAR AND BERRY JUICE

Apples and pears taste sublime when juiced together. Berries are packed with nutrients, especially potassium, and any berries – strawberries, raspberries, blackberries – work well with apple and pear.

2 apples
1 pear
About a dozen berries

Juice all the ingredients, reserving a few pieces of apple to put through the juicer last. This will help flush the thicker berry juice through the machine.

APPLE, WATERCRESS AND LEMON JUICE

This is a great breakfast-time drink that really wakes your whole system up for the day.

2 apples
½ lemon
As much watercress as you like

Put all the ingredients through a juicer. Serve.

FRUIT MEDLEY

This is a great fruit punch. You can use different fruit to suit the season.

½ apple, peeled
½ pear, peeled
1 tangerine
12 grapes
1 peach

Put all the ingredients through a juicer. Serve.

Smoothies

Some fruit requires peeling and seeding due to the toxicity of the skins or seeds. Some examples would be: peel oranges, bananas and grapefruit, kiwi, papaya, and any that have been waxed. Seed apples, peaches, plums, and all other pitted fruit and vegetables.

BANANA AND PINEAPPLE SMOOTHIE

1 banana
2 spears of pineapple
3 tbsp live natural yoghurt

Peel the banana and break into chunks. Remove the pineapple skin and cut into spears then chunks. Put the yoghurt, banana and pineapple into the blender and blend until smooth.

BANANA AND PEACH SMOOTHIE WITH BERRIES

1 banana
2 peaches
12 strawberries, raspberries or blueberries
3 tbsp live natural yoghurt

Peel and cut the banana. Remove the stones from the peaches and cut into chunks. Remove the green stalks from the strawberries. Put all the ingredients into the blender and blend until smooth.

Dressings

LEMON DRESSING FOR FRUIT SALADS

6 lemons
3 tbsp wheat germ oil
2 tsp maple syrup
Pinch of cayenne pepper or cinnamon

Squeeze the lemons and blend the juice with the other
ingredients.

LEMON POPPY SEED DRESSING

This is a light summer dressing for any vegetable salad, or
you can use it as a dip for raw summer vegetables.

2 fl oz light mayonnaise
2 fl oz fat-free sour cream
2 fl oz skimmed or low-fat milk
4 tbsp Xylitol
2 tbsp distilled white vinegar
1 tbsp poppy seeds
1 tsp finely chopped lemon peel

Add all the ingredients to a small bowl and whisk together
until smooth. Cover and keep in the refrigerator until ready
to serve.

LEMON AND OLIVE OIL SALAD DRESSING

½ small garlic clove, finely minced
1 level tsp sea salt
3 tbsp extra virgin olive oil
1 tbsp freshly squeezed lemon juice

In a salad bowl, use the back of a tablespoon to crush the garlic and salt to a paste. Stir in the olive oil and the lemon juice and adjust seasoning to taste.

HUMMUS

1 14.5-oz can of salt- and sugar-free chickpeas, drained
    (save the liquid)
3 tsp lemon juice
3 cloves garlic, peeled
2 tbsp sesame tahini
Pinch of sea salt and black pepper

Add all the ingredients to a food processor and process until smooth. Add the saved liquid until you achieve a spreadable texture.

Soups

PEA AND MUSHROOM SOUP

1 tbsp olive oil
1 onion, chopped
2 garlic cloves, peeled and chopped
1 carrot, chopped
5 oz mushrooms, sliced
1½ pints (24 oz) water or chicken stock
3½ oz split green peas
Pinch of black pepper to taste

Heat the olive oil in a large pan and sauté the onion, garlic, carrot and mushrooms until soft. Add the water or chicken stock and peas. Reduce the heat and simmer for 45 minutes or until the peas are soft. Season to taste.

LENTIL SOUP

Serves 2

Served with whole-grain bread, this is a nutritious and tasty snack.

4 oz red lentils
15 fl oz vegetable stock
15 fl oz water
½ onion
1 garlic clove
½ tsp sunflower oil
Pinch of ground cumin
2 lemon wedges

Pour the lentils into a pan, add the stock and water and bring to the boil. Simmer for 30 minutes, removing any scum that rises to the surface with a wooden spoon.

Peel and chop the onion. Peel and crush the garlic. Heat the oil in a nonstick frying pan over a moderate heat and fry the onion and garlic until the onions have browned.

Add a pinch of ground cumin to the lentils and stir well. Serve the soup in individual bowls and garnish with the onion and garlic mixture and lemon wedges.

VEGETABLE SOUP

Serves 4

4 tbsp extra virgin olive oil
1 large onion, finely chopped
2 garlic cloves, finely chopped
2 large zucchini, trimmed and grated
4 new potatoes, scrubbed and grated
1 large carrot, grated
Vegetables of your choice: 18 oz Brussels sprouts, or
    2 stalks of celery, chopped, or 3 large leeks, chopped,
    or a can of peas, soya beans, or flageolet or great
    northern beans
2½ pints vegetable stock

Heat the oil. Add the onion and garlic and sweat gently for 5 minutes. Add the grated and chopped vegetables (but not the beans, if using) and heat for 5 more minutes, stirring all the time. Pour in the stock and let it simmer for 10 minutes.

Transfer the mixture to a blender until smooth and then return it to the pan. Rinse the beans and peas, if you want to include them, and add to the pan. Bring the soup back to a simmer for 5 minutes before serving.

CARROT SOUP

Serves 4

1 lb carrots
1 small onion
1 tsp sunflower oil
1½ pints vegetable stock
1 orange
1 tbsp chopped coriander

Rinse, peel and chop the carrots and the onion. Heat the oil in a pan, add the onion and fry over a gentle heat for a few minutes. Add the carrots and cook for around 2 minutes. Add the stock, zest and juice of the orange and the coriander. Bring to the boil and leave to simmer with the lid on for about 45 minutes.

Pour the soup into a blender or food processor and process till smooth. Rinse the pan. Return the soup to the pan and heat until very hot. Serve with croutons if desired.

Main meals

CHICKEN GINGER SKEWERS

Serves 2

4 oz skinless organic chicken breasts
4 tbsp plus 2 tsp extra virgin olive oil
4 tbsp plus 2 tsp lemon juice
½ medium garlic clove, crushed
1 tsp fresh ginger, grated
½ tsp ground ginger
3 oz quinoa
Large bunch flat-leaf parsley, coriander, and mint, chopped
6 scallions, sliced
1 lemon, quartered

Soak 4 wooden skewers in water for 10 minutes. Put the chicken into a bowl with 2 tsp extra virgin olive oil, 2 tsp lemon juice, the garlic and fresh and ground ginger and stir to coat the chicken. Leave to marinate for 15 minutes.

Cook the quinoa and allow to cool. Put in a bowl with the chopped herbs, scallions, 4 tbsp extra virgin olive oil and 4 tbsp lemon juice.

Preheat the grill. Skewer the chicken and grill for 3–4 minutes on each side until golden. Divide the quinoa on to 2 plates, top with chicken skewers and serve with lemon quarters.

RISOTTO

Serves 2-4

1 tbsp olive oil
1 medium onion, finely chopped
2–4 skinless chicken breasts, chopped, 2–4 portions of
      seafood of choice or 8–10 oz vegetables (such as
      mushrooms, asparagus, beans), cut into small pieces
Basil or nutmeg (if using chicken)
Lemon juice or thyme (if using seafood or vegetables)
9 oz risotto rice
2 tbsp tomato purée
1 pint stock
2 tbsp (1 oz) grated Cheddar cheese
Parmesan cheese, optional

Gently heat the oil in a pan. If you are using chicken, cook gently until brown, then add the onion and basil or nutmeg and cook for about 5 minutes. If using seafood or vegetables, cook the onion and lemon juice or thyme first for about 5 minutes. Add the seafood or vegetables and stir-fry for a few minutes until cooked. Give it a stir, then add the risotto rice.

Add the tomato purée and stir well before adding the stock. Bring to the boil, then cover and turn the heat to its lowest setting and leave for 15 minutes. This should be enough time to cook the rice; if not, add some water. Stir in the cheese. Allow to stand and cool for a few minutes, then sprinkle with Parmesan cheese if you like and serve.

LEMON, CHICKEN AND BARLEY SALAD

Serves 2

¾ pint filtered water
5 oz uncooked quick-cooking barley
9 oz diced cooked chicken
3½ oz celery, diced
3½ oz tomatoes, chopped
3½ oz red onions, chopped
3½ oz cucumber, sliced
1 tsp olive oil
2 tbsp freshly squeezed lemon juice
1 tsp Dijon mustard
5 lettuce leaves
1 lemon, cut into 6 wedges

Bring the water to a boil in a saucepan, add the barley and return to the boil. Once boiling reduce the heat, cover with a lid and simmer for 10 minutes until the barley is tender, stirring occasionally. Drain any remaining water away and leave to cool slightly. Then, toss the barley with the remaining ingredients, except for the lemon wedges. Serve on lettuce leaves and garnish with the wedges.

OPEN-FACED SANDWICH WITH CUCUMBER AND SMOKED SALMON

1 slice of whole-grain bread
A little soft cheese
2 thin slices of smoked salmon
Cucumber slices
Fresh lemon juice
Freshly ground black pepper
Few sprigs of fresh dill

Spread the bread with a thin layer of soft cheese then top with salmon and cucumber. Drizzle with the juice of 1 lemon, season with black pepper and finish off with a few sprigs of fresh dill.

LEMON-CRUSTED SALMON

Serves 4

4½ oz skinless salmon fillets
2 medium slices of whole-grain bread
2 tbsp freshly chopped coriander
1 tbsp (½ oz) butter, melted
Zest and juice of 1 lemon

Preheat the grill to a medium setting. Season the salmon and place on a foil-lined baking tray.

Put the bread and coriander in a food processor until you have a mixture of fine crumbs. Mix with the melted butter and lemon zest and most of the juice, drizzling the remaining juice over the salmon. Press the crumb crust on to the salmon fillets and grill for 8 minutes until the crust is crisp and the fish is cooked through. Serve with sugar snap peas, new potatoes, and 1 tbsp low-fat mayonnaise.

MARINATED SHRIMP WITH CORN, BEAN AND CHICKPEA SALSA

Serves 4

14-oz can cannellini beans, drained and rinsed
11-oz can sweetcorn, drained and rinsed
10½-oz can chickpeas, drained and rinsed
1 tsp grated lemon zest
2 tbsp chopped coriander leaves
18 oz large, unpeeled, raw shrimp
2 tbsp lemon juice
1 tbsp sesame oil
2 garlic cloves, crushed
2 tsp grated ginger
Extra virgin olive oil spray
Lemon wedges

Combine the cannellini beans, corn, and chickpeas in a large bowl and stir in the lemon zest and coriander. Peel the shrimp, leaving the tails on.

For the marinade, combine the lemon juice, sesame oil, garlic and ginger in a small bowl. Add the shrimp and gently stir to coat them in the marinade. Cover and refrigerate for 3 hours.

Lightly spray a griddle pan with oil and place over a high heat. Add the shrimp and cook for 3–5 minutes until pink and cooked through. Brush the shrimp with marinade while cooking. Serve with the corn, bean and chickpea salsa and wedges of lemon.

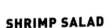

SHRIMP SALAD

Mixed green leaves
Cucumber, sliced
Spring onions, chopped
Cherry tomatoes, halved
Red peppers, thinly sliced
1 tsp extra virgin olive oil
1 tsp lemon juice
1 tsp balsamic vinegar
4½ oz large, cooked, peeled shrimp

Toss as many of the salad ingredients as you would like with olive oil, lemon juice, and vinegar. Arrange on a plate and garnish with shrimp.

TUNA SALAD WITH SOY NUTS

Serves 2

Soy nuts are made from whole soya beans which have been soaked in water and then baked until crisp and brown. Soy nuts are similar in texture and flavor to peanuts.

8 oz canned tuna in water
6 oz shredded carrots
1 oz red onion, sliced
4 oz goat's cheese, cubed
2½ oz soy nuts
2 oz breadcrumbs

Dressing

2 fl oz olive oil
2 tbsp lemon juice
Pinch of black pepper
1 garlic clove, crushed

Put the salad ingredients into a bowl. Mix the dressing ingredients separately. Toss the salad with the dressing and serve.

WARM BEAN SALAD

Serves 2

9 oz okra, finely sliced
2 large garlic cloves, crushed
6 fl oz water
6 oz canned butter beans, drained and rinsed
6 oz canned red kidney beans, drained and rinsed
2 tsp lemon juice
2 tsp extra virgin olive oil
Large handful of mixed herbs, chopped
Black pepper
2 thick slices of crusty bread

Put the okra, garlic and water into a saucepan, cover and bring to the boil. Reduce the heat and simmer gently for 3 minutes until soft. Drain.

Meanwhile, in a separate saucepan, gently heat the beans with the lemon juice. Strain, then add the okra and garlic, olive oil, herbs and pepper to taste. Stir gently and serve with the bread. You could add some chopped tomatoes and red peppers to the finished salad for an extra nutrient shot.

MEXICAN BEAN SALAD

Serves 2

1 cup (8 oz) black-eyed beans, drained
½ cup (4 oz) sweetcorn
Lemon juice dressing (see page 121)
6 oz washed and dried lettuce leaves, torn into
    small pieces
1 fresh tomato, chopped
1 tbsp (1 oz) Cheddar cheese, grated

Mix the beans and sweetcorn with the dressing and leave for an hour or so. Arrange the lettuce on two plates and spoon over the bean mixture. Add the tomato and sprinkle grated cheese on top.

POTATO AND VEGETABLE SALAD

Serves 4

10 new potatoes with skins on
Black pepper and sea salt to taste
2 tbsp extra virgin olive oil
½ cup (4 oz) broccoli
1 medium-sized lettuce, washed and torn into small pieces
½ cup (4 oz) spinach, chopped
3 tbsp (3 oz) alfalfa sprouts
2 tbsp (2 oz) red cabbage, sliced

Mayonnaise with Lemon Juice Dressing

1 large egg
1 tsp Dijon mustard
½ tsp salt
¼ tsp freshly ground white pepper
1½ tsp white wine vinegar
1 cup (8 fl oz) peanut, olive or corn oil
1–2 tbsp lemon juice

Boil the potatoes for approximately 20 minutes until tender.
Drain, cool and cut into chunks. Put in a bowl, add pepper,
salt and oil and toss well. Place the potatoes on greaseproof
paper and bake at 400°F for 10 minutes.

Wash the broccoli and cut into bite-sized florets, discarding the stalks. Steam the broccoli for a few minutes until tender. Plunge it into cold water for about a minute to prevent it overcooking and drain well.

Place the lettuce and spinach in a bowl and add the alfalfa sprouts and red cabbage. Cut the broccoli lengthwise and add to the greens.

To make the mayonnaise with lemon juice dressing, place everything but the oil and lemon juice in the blender or processor container. Process for 5 seconds in the blender or for 15 seconds in the processor. With the motor running, add the oil, first in a drizzle, then in a thin, steady stream. When all the oil has been added, stop the motor and taste. Add the lemon juice. If the sauce is too thick, thin with hot water or lemon juice. If it is too thin, process a little longer.

Remove the potatoes from the oven and add to the salad.

ZUCCHINI AND RICOTTA SALAD

Serves 2

4 medium zucchini
Extra virgin olive oil
Freshly ground black pepper
5 oz ricotta
¾ oz shaved pecorino cheese
½ oz fresh basil leaves, torn
½ oz fresh mint leaves, torn
Juice of 2 lemons
Green leafy salad
Handful of mixed nuts and seeds

Cut the zucchini into rounds about ⅛ in thick. Heat a non-stick frying pan, brush the zucchini with oil on both sides and cook in batches until golden brown; season with freshly ground black pepper.

Put the first batch of zucchini into the bottom of a broad, shallow bowl. Top with some crumbled ricotta, pecorino and herbs plus some lemon juice and extra virgin olive oil. Keep layering them up like this until you have used them all.

Finish by adding some herbs and drizzle with some extra virgin olive oil and a little lemon juice. Serve with a green leafy salad and a handful of mixed nuts and seeds.

VEGETABLE STEW

Serves 2–4

1 large onion, chopped
1 large garlic clove, peeled and chopped
1 tbsp olive oil
6 oz fresh spinach, chopped
14 oz can of salt- and sugar-free chickpeas
14 oz can of salt-free tomatoes, chopped
4 or 5 fresh tomatoes, chopped
½ cup (2½ oz) raisins
2 new potatoes, peeled and chopped
3 oz brown rice
Lemon juice and black pepper to taste

Fry the onion and garlic in the olive oil. Add the spinach and cook until limp then stir in the rest of the ingredients, except the black pepper and lemon juice. Cook for 45 minutes or until the potato is soft when pricked by a fork. You may need to add a little water if the stew gets too thick. Add lemon juice and black pepper, and serve.

PASTA SALAD

Serves 2

This makes a good snack salad. It can easily be packed into a container and taken with you to work.

¼ lb whole-wheat pasta
½ tbsp olive oil
½ onion, diced
½ garlic clove, crushed
2 tbsp tomato purée
1½ tsp (½ oz) basil leaves, chopped

Cook the pasta as directed on the package. Meanwhile, heat the oil in a pan, add the onion and garlic and fry until the onion is soft. Stir in the tomato purée and basil. Drain the pasta, combine with the onion mixture and leave to cool. Serve chilled.

EGG AND SPINACH CAKE

Serves 4

¼ risotto rice
½ tsp sunflower oil
1 small onion, finely chopped
¼ lb frozen spinach (defrosted)
2 eggs
¼ cup (2 oz) freshly grated Parmesan cheese
Pinch of cayenne pepper

Cook the rice according to the packet instructions.

Meanwhile, heat the oil in a pan, add the onion and fry until light brown. Put the spinach, rice and onion in a bowl. In another bowl, crack the eggs and lightly beat the whites and yokes together. Add the eggs, cheese and pepper to the spinach, rice and onion mixture and stir thoroughly. Transfer to a cake pan and bake for about half an hour in a hot oven approximately 200°F.

Desserts and Snacks

FRUIT KEBABS WITH LEMON CREAM

1 small container (6 oz) natural yoghurt
2 tbsp low-fat soft cheese
1 tsp poppy seeds
½ tsp grated lemon peel
2 tbsp lemon juice
Fruit: strawberries, cantaloupe, kiwi, etc.

Combine the yoghurt with the soft cheese, blending till smooth. Stir in the poppy seeds, lemon peel and lemon juice. Refrigerate for two hours to allow the flavors to blend. Thread fruit onto toothpicks or skewers and serve with the sauce.

DRIED FRUIT COMPOTE

Serves 2

1½ tbsp (1 oz) dried figs
1½ tbsp (1 oz) dried apricots
1½ tbsp (1 oz) dried prunes
1½ tbsp (1 oz) dried apple
1½ tbsp (1 oz) raisins
3½ fl oz apple juice

Put the dried fruit into a bowl with the apple juice and leave in the fridge overnight. Serve chilled.

BAKED APPLES WITH STUFFING

Serves 2

2 good-sized cooking apples
Stuffing suggestions: dates, cinnamon, raisins, almonds
1 tbsp maple syrup

Core the apples and slit the skins in a ring around the middle. Stuff with chosen filling and maple syrup. Bake at 350°F for 45 minutes to 1 hour or until the fruit is tender. Serve hot or cold.

BANANA SURPRISE

Serves 2

2 bananas
1½ tbsp (1 oz) chopped dates
1½ tbsp (1 oz) chopped dried apricots
1½ tbsp (1 oz) seedless grapes
1½ tbsp (1 oz) chopped almonds

Mash the bananas in a bowl and stir in the fruit and nuts. Spread the mixture in a freezer tray and freeze for 2 hours. Serve chilled.

FRUIT AND RYVITA DESSERT

Serves 6

2 bananas
2 apples
8 dried apricots
8–12 Ryvita crackers
¼ cup (2 oz) broken walnuts

Prepare the fruit, cut into small pieces and put into a saucepan. Add a few tbsp water and simmer for 10 minutes or until the fruit is soft, adding more water if the mixture becomes too dry.

Put the crackers into the bottom of your dessert bowls – you may have to break them to make them fit. When the fruit is soft, pour over the crackers. Serve with a sprinkling of walnuts.

FRUIT AND NUT SALAD

Serves 4

1 peach, sliced
2 oranges, peeled, deseeded and sliced
8 oz fresh pineapple, chopped
6 oz seedless grapes
2 tbsp (1 oz) brazil nuts, chopped
Juice of 1 lemon
Handful of toasted almonds

Put the peach and orange slices into four serving bowls. Mix the pineapple, grapes and brazil nuts and place on top of the peach and orange slices. Spoon over the lemon juice and sprinkle with toasted almonds.

RED FRUIT DESSERT

Serves 2

½ cup (4 oz) strawberries
½ cup (4 oz) raspberries
2 tbsp (2 oz) red currants
2 fl oz unsweetened cranberry or apple juice

Remove leaves and stems and wash the fruit under cold, running water. Put the fruit into a bowl and stir in the cranberry or apple juice. Chill for half an hour and serve with low-fat yoghurt or vanilla ice cream.

LEMON ALMOND CAKE

Serves 1 or more!

¼ lb (4 oz) unsalted butter at room temperature
3½ oz light brown sugar
1 tbsp lemon zest
1 tsp vanilla extract
1 tsp baking powder
½ tsp sea salt
3 egg yolks and 4 egg whites
3½ oz ground almonds
2½ oz plain flour
3 fl oz lemon juice
½ tsp cream of tartar
Xylitol, optional

Preheat the oven to 350°F.

Butter an 8 inch-round cake pan. Line the bottom of the pan with waxed paper and butter the paper. Lightly flour the pan, being sure to tap out any excess flour.

Beat the butter with brown sugar, lemon zest, vanilla, baking powder and salt until light and fluffy. Add the egg yolks one by one, beating well each time. Combine the ground almonds and flour and stir into the egg yolks, together with the lemon juice.

Whip the egg whites with the cream of tartar until they form soft peaks. Fold the egg whites into the batter in 3 batches. Spoon the batter into the prepared cake pan and bake for approximately 35–40 minutes or until a pale golden color and a skewer comes out clean. Leave to cool on a wire rack for 15 minutes. Remove the cake from the pan and peel off the paper. Let the cake cool completely before transferring to a platter and dusting with Xylitol (if desired).

LEMON RECIPES FOR BEAUTY

Long before our bathroom cabinets were filled with commercial beauty products, our ancestors made use of natural ingredients, such as the lemon, for a wide range of hair and body treatments. Lemon can cleanse, tone and firm your skin in the most natural way possible, which is why you will often find it as an ingredient in cosmetics.

You can use lemons to create safe and effective home beauty treatments to lighten, exfoliate and tone skin and to invigorate your spirit. Try some of the beauty recipes that follow. If you aren't convinced, try rinsing your face in lemon water just before you go to bed, and notice how fresh and soft your skin feels the next day.

FACEMASK FOR NORMAL OR OILY SKIN

1 small banana
1 tsp honey
8 drops of lemon juice (more if you prefer)

Mash the banana and mix with the other ingredients. Apply to a clean face and leave for about 5–10 minutes. Remove with warm water and apply toner and moisturizer.

FACEMASK TO REDUCE APPEARANCE OF LINES

1 egg yolk
1 tbsp jojoba oil
Juice of 1 lemon

Blend the egg yolk and jojoba oil. Squeeze the lemon and add the juice to the blend. Massage into the skin and leave for 20 minutes. Remove with cold water.

FACEMASK FOR DRY SKIN

1 ripe banana
3 drops lemon essential oil
2 egg yolks
1 tbsp jojoba oil
1 tbsp avocado oil
2 lemons

Mash the banana and blend with the rest of the ingredients, except the lemons, into a smooth paste. Apply to skin and leave for 20 minutes. Rinse with the juice of 2 lemons added to 1¾ pints of warm water.

CLEANSING SOLUTION

1 lemon
3 fl oz milk
1 tbsp honey

Squeeze the lemon and mix the juice into the milk, adding the honey. Using a cotton wool ball, gently dab the mixture over your skin and leave for 2 minutes. Then rinse your face with clean, warm water.

LEMON JUICE ASTRINGENT

Squeeze some lemon juice into a glass jar. Dab some on to your face every morning, let it set for 10 minutes, then wash it off with warm water followed by a moisturizer.

ROUGH SKIN

If you have rough skin on your knees or elbows squeeze the juice of 2 to 3 lemons into 1 pint of warm water and add 2 tbsp of runny honey. Soak a cotton wool pad in this solution and apply to rough skin. If your hands or feet feel rough, soak them in the solution.

DISCOLOURED ELBOWS

To lighten discolored elbows: cut a lemon in half and place an elbow in each half for approximately 10 minutes. The lemon acids will gently break down the dark patches of skin so they may be washed away.

TO EXFOLIATE AND LIGHTEN SKIN

To exfoliate dead skin and diminish the appearance of freckles and age spots, gently rub a cut lemon and ½ tsp sugar granules over the skin for a few minutes. Repeat at least once a week until the darkened areas fade. Another way to lighten age spots is to simply sit with a slice of lemon applied directly to the area for 10 minutes. Repeat once a week until the spots fade.

NAIL PROBLEMS

If your nails are stained or weak, apply some lemon juice mixed with water after washing them. Leave it on for a few minutes. If you do this frequently, it will help your nails look healthier and shiny.

NATURAL HIGHLIGHTS

Lemon can help you to create highlights in your hair during summer. However, lemons dry out the hair so be careful not to use this recipe too often. Prepare a cup with warm water and lemon juice (about 1 lemon should be enough, depending on the length of your hair). After shampooing, simply apply the lemon water to the hair and leave it on in the sunshine for a few hours (making sure you wear sunblock).

LEMON HAIR CONDITIONER

To add bounce and shine, mix the juice of 1 lemon with 1 cup of warm water and apply to the hair. Leave it on for a few minutes, then rinse.

DANDRUFF TREATMENT

Mix a few tbsp of fresh lemon juice with warm olive oil and rub gently into the scalp. Leave it on for 15 minutes, then shampoo and rinse as usual.

FOR SMOOTH, PRETTY FEET

In a foot bath, combine:

1 cup (8 fl oz) lemon juice
2 tbsp olive oil
3½ fl oz milk
Enough water to fill the basin
You may also add a few drops of your favorite essential oil
for fragrance, if you like

Soak your feet for 15 minutes then rinse with warm water.
Do this once a week for several weeks for noticeably softer,
smoother feet.

LEMON BATH

Bathing with lemon juice is a wonderful way to spoil yourself; in the rising steam you get the uplifting scent of the
essential oils, while the lemon juice rejuvenates your skin.
Squeeze the juice out of 5 lemons and stir into your warm
bath with 8 drops of lemon essential oil and 3½ pints of whey
or buttermilk. Relax for 15 minutes, and let your body and
mind soak in all that goodness.

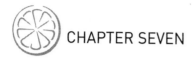 CHAPTER SEVEN

The Lemon Juice Diet Exercise Plan for Weight Loss

Exercise is an essential part of the Lemon Juice Diet because it's a fantastic way to boost your metabolism and aid digestion, making weight loss efficient. But before you start worrying about all the sweating and hard work you need to do – relax. This exercise plan is really straight-forward, based on walking and a few abdominal exercises. You just need some well-fitting sneakers and space in your living room to do some toning and stretching. It's that simple.

Note

If you are overweight, have high blood pressure or a pre-existing medical condition make sure you check with your doctor before beginning an exercise regime. Once you know it is safe to exercise, do so safely. There shouldn't be any pain, discomfort, shortness of breath or dizziness. If things don't feel right, stop immediately and talk to your doctor.

EXERCISE, DIGESTION AND WEIGHT LOSS

As far as weight loss and your health are concerned, the more active you are the better. Exercise reduces your risk of heart disease and boosts your mood and energy levels. It increases the rate at which you burn calories for up to 12 hours, so you're burning more calories even while you are resting, making your body more likely to draw in nutrients from your food and supplements. Taking regular exercise also builds muscle power, and muscles are fat-burning machines.

Another great plus is that exercise improves your circulation. It speeds up the natural detoxification and elimination process that is essential for weight loss. When you exercise, you breathe more deeply. The diaphragm – a dome-shaped muscle that separates your chest and abdominal cavity – is pulled down to allow for deeper inhalation, and relaxes as you exhale. This action massages the digestive tract and promotes regular bowel movements. Finally, exercise also encourages you to drink more water, which is important for healthy digestion and weight loss.

So, if you want improved digestion, natural weight loss and more energy, you need to make a commitment to exercise every single day, even if it's just to go out for a 30-minute walk.

TIME TO GET WALKING

A regular walking program, combined with the Lemon Juice Diet, is one of the best ways to improve your digestion and kick-start weight loss. Walking results in the rhythmic contraction and relaxation of muscles as well as rhythmic pressure changes in body cavities that can improve blood circulation and, by so doing, gently and effectively aid digestion and weight loss. And not only does walking encourage the body to shed fat, it also helps build muscle, strengthen bones and boost circulation. In short, if you've got weight to lose and want to look toned with glowing skin, walking is great! It's safe and you can do it any time, anywhere. All you need is a pair of walking shoes and some motivation!

Now it's time to get moving. Instead of driving around the car park for ages to get the spot next to the door, park farther away and walk. Stop taking elevators and escalators, and use the stairs. Instead of slumping in front of the television at home, put your coat or jacket on and get some fresh air. If it's raining outside, don't let that stop you; take an umbrella. If the weather is really bad, put on your favorite music and dance instead. Okay, this isn't walking, but it's still moving energetically, and the more you move and breathe deeply the better. Another great option is to buy a small trampoline and do some gentle bouncing while you watch your favourite program.

Good Walking Technique

A humble walk can easily be turned into a fat-burning and muscle-building workout that can tone your buttocks, hips and thighs. Putting one foot in front of the other is easy, but to get the most from your workout you need to make sure you walk correctly.

- Sort your posture out first by relaxing your shoulders, gently pulling in your tummy and lifting your ribcage slightly.
- Look forwards, not down, with your chin up and parallel to the ground.
- Relax your arms, keeping them close to your body.
- With each step, land on your heel and then transfer your weight to the ball of your foot, rolling forward in a smooth heel-to-toe movement.
- Try to walk briskly, at a pace that leaves you feeling breathless but comfortable. You should still be able to talk in short sentences.
- Walk faster by taking quicker, not bigger, steps as unnaturally long strides will throw your posture out of alignment.
- Your movement should be fluid, so don't bounce.

If you're a beginner, walk at a moderate pace first; this should feel slightly challenging as if you are walking with intent, not just taking a gentle stroll. When you feel more confident, go at a faster pace, pushing yourself a bit beyond your comfort zone. When you feel really confident walk at speed; this pace should feel like you are walking as fast as you can, making sure you maintain correct posture and technique. Adding even a slight incline to your walking route will make a real difference to the intensity of your workout, so find a hill to walk up, or if you're using a treadmill, up the gradient on that. The trick is to keep your pace constant, whether you're walking uphill or down, as this will maintain a steady heart rate and maximum calorie burning.

You need some comfortable but supportive shoes or sneakers and loose-fitting clothing. Your footwear should feel roomy around the toes, give good heel cushioning and be comfy and light. Different shoes provide varying degrees of support, so if you are unsure, ask for advice in your local sports shop.

Your Walking Workout Plan

Your walking workout plan will help you burn fat and boost your confidence, stamina and energy levels. Warm up by walking at a moderate pace for five minutes and then start setting a brisker pace. Up your speed when you don't feel challenged and reduce it when you feel tired. A good tip is to swing your arms as you walk faster, until you are about to break into a run, then take this down a few notches so you can maintain it. Five minutes before you end your workout, slow to a moderate pace again to help you cool down.

Be careful not to launch yourself into a vigorous work-out plan if you haven't exercised for a while or have a lot of weight to lose. Instead, start slowly and build up, and gradually increase the intensity and length of your workout when you feel you have more stamina.

For example, in week one you could walk slowly for five minutes, then build up to five minutes of walking at moderate pace, and then cool down for five minutes by walking moderately again, so that your daily walking workout is 15 minutes. Then in week two, add five minutes to the time you walk at moderate pace so you are walking for a total of 20 minutes a day. The week after, you could build this up to 25 minutes so that by week four you have hit your target of 30 minutes' walking a day.

If you feel up to it, you can then think about increasing to 45 minutes or doing 25 minutes at a faster pace or at speed, but if you simply haven't the time, sticking with 30 minutes at moderate pace is fine as long as you push yourself to work hard in each workout. Two or three days a week you could also split your walk in half by, for example, walking for 15 minutes before work and then 15 minutes in your lunch hour.

Power Walking Workout Plan

Week 1
1 x 20-minute moderate-pace walk
2 x 30-minute moderate-pace walks
1 x 45-minute moderate-pace walk
1 x 15-minute walk at speed
1 x 20-minute faster-pace walk
1 rest day

Week 2
3 x 30-minute moderate-pace walks
2 x 40-minute moderate-pace walks
1 x 25-minute faster-pace walk
1 rest day

Week 3
2 x 30-minute moderate-pace walks
3 x 40-minute moderate-pace walks
1 x 30-minute faster-pace walk
1 rest day

Week 4
2 x 30-minute moderate-pace walks
2 x 40-minute moderate-pace walks
1 x 30-minute faster-pace walk
1 x 25-minute walk at speed
1 rest day

Troubleshooting

As you start your walking workout plan you may experience a few aches and pains. This is normal if you are new to exercise.

To Avoid Knee Pain

Sit on the floor with your right leg stretched out in front of you and your left leg bent with your foot on the floor. Put your hands behind you and sit up straight. With your right foot flexed, lift your left leg a few inches off the floor, hold for a few seconds and then lower. Do five lifts and then shift to the other leg. Do this two to four times a week.

To Avoid Calf Pain

Before and after your workout, face a wall, tree or post and press both palms against it. Keep your left foot on the floor and bend your left knee. Press the heel of your right foot into the floor until you feel a gentle stretch in your calf. Now change legs.

To Avoid Arm Pain

Stretch your upper body before each walk by standing with your feet shoulder width apart and raising your right arm over your head, bending at the elbow so your right hand is behind your head. Place your left hand over your right elbow and gently pull the elbow to your left, allowing your upper body to bend slightly to the left. Hold for a few deep breaths, release and repeat on the other side.

To Avoid Shin Pain

Stand with your feet almost together and roll up onto your toes, hold for two seconds and then roll back. Then roll onto the outside of your feet and hold for two seconds and back again. Then roll onto your heels with your toes off the ground, hold for two seconds and roll back. Do this routine before you walk as many times as you like.

ANY ACTIVITY COUNTS

If you find it hard to carve 30 minutes of walking time out of your day, your exercise can be spread throughout the day and include activities such as climbing stairs, gardening or cleaning the house. Three 10-minute walks may work better for you than 30 minutes in one go. Any activity counts. Just try to get 30 minutes minimum a day, every day. If you don't think you are getting 30 minutes, find ways to get there by carrying the shopping, walking around the block, washing your car by hand or signing up to a dance class. In the long run, these simple changes can help you lose weight.

Enjoy it!

Whatever activity you choose – be it walking, jogging, dancing, horse riding, stepping, trampolining, swimming, cycling or fencing – make sure it is something you enjoy. Studies show that exercise dropouts are people who punish themselves with routines they dread, so find something you enjoy and stick to it. And if you skip a workout one day, don't let that derail your exercise plan. If you're exercising for 30 minutes a day, giving yourself a day or two off now and again won't hurt.

If you have the time and energy you can challenge yourself, for example by increasing your walking routine to a 30-minute brisk walk before breakfast and a 30-minute walk just before lunch. There's absolutely no reason why you can't do more than 30 minutes of activity a day if you want to, and this will really rev up your metabolism. Do be sensible, though. Overdoing exercise and exercising for more than one and a half or two hours a day is obsessive and unnecessary, unless you are an athlete, dancer or body builder. The important thing is always to make sure you enjoy your exercise and that it improves the quality of your life, but doesn't take over.

TONING AND STRETCHING

Once you have got into the routine of exercising for 30 minutes a day, you should start to think about including some weight-bearing exercises three or four times a week for 10–15 minutes. This is because the more muscle you have, the more calories you will burn and the better your blood sugar balance. You may want to join a gym and use the machines, but if you aren't into these, find ways to use your muscles more in daily life: carry your luggage; do some sit-ups and push-ups when you watch television or some buttock squeezes when you are standing at the bus stop; lift your kids; buy an exercise DVD and do the toning exercises, and so on.

Daily stretching is also a good idea as it will improve your posture, protect your joints from injury and keep you feeling flexible. Great times to have a good stretch are first thing in the morning, last thing at night, after a bath and before and after exercise. It doesn't have to be anything complicated or involve painful yoga poses. Simple stretches, such as standing on your toes and reaching as hard as you can to the ceiling, are highly effective. Don't make the mistake of bouncing when you stretch, though, and gently hold your stretched position for about 30 seconds before relaxing.

Abdominal Exercises

To trim your waistline, traditional toning exercises for the stomach – such as sit-ups and crunches – are good, but there are other kinds of abdominal exercises that can help stimulate your digestion and massage the organs in the abdominal region. The following traditional Chinese exercises can all help improve sluggish digestion and encourage weight loss quickly, easily and safely – without pills, potions or preparation.

The Abdominal Lift

This first exercise should only be done on an empty stomach and is best performed first thing in the morning before breakfast. It prepares your digestive organs for food by giving your entire abdominal area an invigorating massage.

1. Stand with your feet about shoulder width apart. Place your hands just above your knees, with your fingers on the inside of your thighs, right hand on right thigh and left hand on left thigh.
2. Exhale deeply through your mouth till your lungs are empty. Immediately, and without breathing in, use your abdominal muscles to lift your abdomen up and towards your spine as high as you can. Hold the position for 5–10 seconds. Don't breathe in yet!
3. Relax your abdominal wall and let everything fall gently back into place, then take a slow, deep breath (or two).
4. Start by doing two or three rounds and build up to six rounds. As you finish your last round, stand fully upright, arms hanging loosely by your sides.
5. To finish, take a slow, deep breath as you raise your (straight) arms in front of your body and above your head. Stretch up as high as you comfortably can, and hold your breath for a few seconds. Feel your abs stretching.
6. Gently exhale as you slowly and smoothly bring your arms back down to your sides.

Back Twist
Once you've spent a few minutes doing abdominal lifting, do the back twist. This classic Chinese exercise also stimulates your abdominal and digestive organs by massaging them as you twist your torso from side to side.

1. Stand with your back straight and your feet parallel, about shoulder width apart. Bend your knees slightly, sink your weight into your legs and let your arms hang loosely by your sides.

2. Gently twist your upper body and head to the right until you are looking directly behind you. Just let your arms hang loosely and go where they will, but keep your legs and feet pointing ahead throughout the whole exercise; it's your upper body and arms that move.

3. Slowly turn back towards the front and continue around to the left until you are once again looking directly behind you. Continue twisting back and forth from side to side.

4. Remember to let your arms move naturally as you turn. Don't pause at any stage of the exercise. Gradually build up speed and twist in your hips and upper body. Your arms will begin to swing out wide and your hands will slap your sides as you twist.

5. Do 10–15 twists per side. Build up to 30 per side or simply do the exercise for a couple of minutes at a time. When you've finished, don't suddenly stop; gradually slow down and return to the starting position, letting your arms swing until they eventually fall naturally by your sides again. Take a few slow, deep breaths.

Stomach Massage

Massaging your abdomen after meals may improve digestion and absorption of nutrients. In China people often walk very slowly after meals and rub their abdomen at the same time.

1. Stand with your feet parallel and about shoulder width apart.
2. Bend your legs slightly and sink your weight down into them.
3. Keep your back straight or sit on a firm but comfortable straight-backed chair.
4. Rub your hands together briskly until they are hot. Lift any clothing that covers your stomach and place your hands one on top of the other, just below your belly button.
5. Using your palm and fingers rub in small, counter-clockwise circles around your belly button, following the path of your colon, from right to left side. Use fairly firm pressure, but not so much that it's uncomfortable.
6. Rub in small circles at first. Gradually make them bigger so that eventually you are massaging your entire abdominal and stomach area.
7. Focus your attention on the heat penetrating your abdomen.
8. Do 40–50 circles or simply massage for several minutes, once or twice a day.

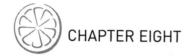 CHAPTER EIGHT

Staying Motivated

In the first week or so of the Lemon Juice Diet your body will be adjusting to the new foods you are eating, and there may well be times when you feel like throwing in the towel. In this chapter you'll find some great advice to help you navigate those 'I'm starving and need something now' or 'I can't be bothered with all this' moments. There are also tips on coping with stress, eating out and what to do if you hit a weight-loss plateau.

WHEN FOOD CRAVINGS STRIKE

Throw Out the Junk
The first thing you can do to help yourself resist temptation is to go through your kitchen cupboards and fridge and throw out all the foods you know aren't good for you. Get rid

of any cakes, biscuits, sweets, potato chips, pies, pastries and so on, as these foods are extremely hard to resist when they are so easily accessible.

You crave the foods you are used to eating, so if you can change what you eat you can weaken your old cravings and strengthen new ones. The first few days will be the toughest and you probably can't eliminate your old cravings completely; but the longer you avoid your trigger foods, the less likely you are to want them. In fact, you may start to crave the fresh and healthy foods you eat, which is a real bonus.

Keep on Drinking Lemon Juice

Have plenty of fresh lemons to hand so you can make up a glass of warm lemon juice anytime, anywhere. Lemon water or tea is a wonderful appetite suppressant. Just squeeze the juice in and throw in the wedge of lemon as well. Drinking a glass of lemon water before you eat can curb food cravings because you feel fuller. And drinking more water can also have a direct impact on energy – you may be reaching for a sugar fix when what you really need to do is rehydrate your body.

Go to Bed Early

Try to get some early nights because sleep will help maintain your energy levels and control your appetite. To get a better night's sleep, try adding some relaxing essential oils like vanilla to your bath or putting a few drops on your pillow. A good night's sleep is important because lack of sleep disrupts hormones, triggering changes in metabolism and an increase in appetite. Tiredness triggers food cravings, so take a power nap for no longer than 20 minutes instead of reaching for the cookie jar.

Eat Little and Often
Remember, if you don't leave more than three hours between meals you simply won't have time to get hungry. The ideal meal plan is to have three balanced meals and two snacks a day. Great healthy snacks include:

- 2 tbsp (1 oz) of either almonds, pecans, or walnuts
- 4½ oz of low-fat yoghurt
- A helping of raw vegetables such as celery, carrots, broccoli, or cauliflower florets

For more snack suggestions, see Meal Plans in Chapter 4.

Ruin Temptation
If you've succumbed to temptation and bought a food that you know isn't good for you, have a small bite and destroy the rest. Don't just throw it in the bin, ruin it; run water over it. You will feel a sense of accomplishment that you are in control of your cravings and not the other way round. Don't think about the money you have wasted; if you don't destroy the temptation, it will end up on your hips.

Slow Down!
When you eat quickly, you end up ingesting more food before your body has a chance to figure out that it's satisfied (not

full). This strategy sounds simple, but it's harder than you think when grabbing a snack or eating on the go has become commonplace. If you take time over your meals, and really chew your food and taste what you are eating, you're less likely to overeat. Put your knife and fork down between bites. And don't forget to wait 20 minutes when you have eaten your meal and want to eat more to see if you are still hungry. Your brain lags behind your stomach by about 15–20 minutes and you may find that you aren't hungry after all.

Enjoy Chocolate

Every evening, eat one delicious, exquisite piece of high-quality, 70-percent-cocoa chocolate. Savor that chocolate. Sit down, relax and do nothing but enjoy the flavor, texture and experience of eating it. Eat slowly, enjoying every bite. And whatever you do, don't feel guilty. A small portion of your favorite food will stop you feeling deprived.

Go for a Walk

When you get a food craving, go for a walk. Exercise is a fantastic appetite suppressant. If walking isn't an option, listen to your favorite music; this will take your mind off eating. Simply listening to a few minutes of upbeat music has been shown to distract people from hunger pangs.

Look in the Mirror

Hang a mirror opposite your seat at the table. One study found that eating in front of mirrors reduced the amount

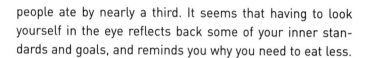

people ate by nearly a third. It seems that having to look yourself in the eye reflects back some of your inner standards and goals, and reminds you why you need to eat less.

Portion Out Your Snack Foods
Don't eat out of the bag or container. Take the food out and put it in a bowl. That way you can see exactly how much you're eating. As an example, divide a 10 oz bag of nuts into 10 small plastic bags. Make sure you eat only one bag at a sitting, and put the rest away where you can't see them. One of the best snacks for beating cravings is a handful of nuts (6 walnuts, 12 almonds or 20 peanuts) with two glasses of water because the protein will keep you feeling satisfied while also giving your taste buds a treat and your energy levels a boost.

Don't Shop on an Empty Stomach
Shopping when you are hungry is a bad idea as it makes you far more likely to binge on calorie-rich, sugary, fatty foods. Make a list of exactly what you need and stick to it. Buy enough vegetables to last for a week. Avoid bargain buying – large-sized packages aren't a bargain if they cost you a new pair of jeans!

Other Tips
- Sniff a lemon, banana, apple, peppermint or vanilla essence. Research from the Smell and Taste Research Foundation in Chicago found that the more frequently people sniffed, the less hungry they were. One theory is

that sniffing food tricks the brain into thinking you are actually eating it. Vanilla essence seems to have appetite-suppressing effects.

- Fresh mint tea is soothing and refreshing. Put a handful of mint leaves in a mug, add boiling water and allow the leaves to steep for a few moments. Other good teas that can help suppress your appetite are lemon, chamomile and verbena.
- If food cravings are intense, you might not be eating enough satisfying and filling foods. Add some more potato or whole-grain pasta or rice to provide bulk to your diet.
- If only chocolate will do, it's a craving, not hunger, so find ways to distract yourself. Phone a friend, write in your journal, or read a book. Cravings typically last 10 minutes, so try to divert your mind and ride it out.
- Brush your teeth early. For whatever reason, when your teeth feel clean you are unlikely to want to eat, so if you get a food craving, brush your teeth or, if that isn't possible, suck on some peppermint.
- Eat vegetables or soup before the main course. This will fill you up and stop you eating too much of the main course.
- Turn off the television or computer while eating, otherwise because of the distraction, your plate might be clean before you realize you've eaten a meal.
- Try to sit down to dinner as a family. The focus on conversation and the day's events helps you to eat less, relax and savor your dinner.

DEALING WITH STRESS

It's also important to look at the impact that stress is having on your diet. Your stomach and intestines are extremely sensitive to stress, and when you feel stressed, digestion shuts down to help your body focus on preparing the fight-or-flight response. This means that food is only partially digested, leading to nutrient deficiency, which as you know by now isn't going to help you lose weight. If stress is long term, your body becomes chronically unable to digest your food, setting you up for weight gain, food cravings, stomach upsets, mood swings and lowered immunity.

Since stress is a huge trigger for cravings, unhealthy eating and weight gain – particularly around the waist – learning to deal with it could potentially save you hundreds of calories a day. This will take some practice. You can try deep breathing or visualizing a serene scene on your own, or you can speed things up by buying a relaxation CD that teaches progressive muscle relaxation.

Plan Ahead

Diet can play a significant role in improving your emotional and physical well-being. If you think about it, we all tend to 'self-medicate' – grabbing a bar of chocolate or another cup of coffee when we feel stressed or a glass of wine when we want to calm down. Planning what you are going to eat in advance can help you at those times when you know you are most vulnerable. Plan your daily eating schedule and know what you will eat for your mid-morning and mid-afternoon snacks. Without planning, you are far more likely to grab something unhealthy.

However much you plan ahead, things sometimes change, so you may have to adapt your eating routine to accommodate stressful situations like work deadlines, rush hour traffic, PMS, family dinners and so on. Keep your cupboards, fridge and freezer well stocked with emergency healthy foods like soup, beans and, of course, plenty of fresh fruit and vegetables and nuts and seeds to nibble on whenever you feel hungry.

Keep to the Lemon Juice Diet

Following the Lemon Juice Diet is the best way to stress-proof your diet. Eating healthy meals and snacks every few hours and ditching caffeine, sugar and alcohol will keep your blood sugar levels stable and give you the nutrients you need to feel calm and stable during times of crisis. Boosting your magnesium intake by eating more green vegetables, nuts, seeds, whole grains and legumes will help. Magnesium is building itself a reputation as the calming mineral because it is used by the body to make energy, balance blood sugar levels and maintain healthy blood pressure, all things that can go haywire under stress. Other stress-busting nutrients are vitamin B5 found in eggs, fish, lentils, soya and whole grains, and vitamin C found in berries, broccoli, cabbage, peppers, kale and citrus fruit, like lemon.

Cut Down on Caffeine

It's also a good idea to make sure you don't drink coffee before 10am. The ideal is to drink none at all but if that is too stressful have one or two a day, but never on an empty stomach. Getting a caffeine fix when your body is still waking up becomes another form of stress; what's more, your body becomes immune to the caffeine and needs more for it to have an effect.

Have Your Oats

After your vitamin C boost with a glass of lemon juice in the morning try to eat oats for breakfast because these versatile whole grains are loaded with B vitamins and magnesium, and the milk will help the amino acid tryptophan cross into the nervous system where it is used to make serotonin, the feel-good hormone. Other foods that raise serotonin levels include bananas, yoghurt, figs and dates.

Go Easy on the Exercise

Intense workouts raise levels of the stress hormone cortisol so if you are drained by long-term stress, don't make things worse. Take your training down a notch – try walking, gentle swimming or yoga rather than a hard-core aerobic marathon.

EATING OUT

We all dine out these days and although this means you have less control over what you eat, it's still possible to make healthy choices. Chinese, Japanese, Thai or Malaysian menus tend to be healthier but this doesn't mean you can't eat Italian, French, Mexican, Indian or other foods. You just need to know what to order. Here are some helpful tips:

- Don't arrive starving at the restaurant; have a light snack an hour or so before.
- Avoid the bread basket and stick to water or a dish of olives before your food arrives.
- Watch out for hidden sugar and fat in sauces, dressings and dips – ask for them to be served on the side so you're in control of how much goes on your food.
- If you're not very hungry or would like to eat less, try ordering a couple of small starters, or a starter and a salad, instead of a main course.
- It's best to stick with water as your beverage, skipping the coffee and alcohol if possible. If you'd like a drink with more flavor, try sparkling mineral water with a slice of lemon or lime.
- Soups make great starters as most are fairly low in calories, but soups with a cream base are higher in calories and fat.
- Look for foods that are grilled, baked, poached or steamed. These cooking methods use fewer fats and oils and are generally much lower in calories. You want

to avoid deep-fried foods, but it's not always easy to tell. In general, stay away from anything described as 'crispy,' and ask if you're not sure. In Asian restaurants, choose steamed brown rice and noodles instead of fried versions.

- Grilled fish and vegetables are very healthy choices. You can go one step further and request that the food be grilled without butter or oil.
- Foods containing whole grains, like whole-wheat bread and brown rice dishes, are also healthier alternatives.
- Choose a baked potato or steamed vegetables instead of chips or fried vegetables. Always order some vegetable dishes, whether it's a salad or a side dish of green beans or broccoli. If you haven't had enough vegetables, order some more.
- Enjoy pasta? Avoid cream-based sauces that are high in fat and calories. Opt instead for tomato-based sauces such as marinara, which can even be counted towards your vegetable intake!
- If you order a pudding, either choose something low in fat with berries and fruit, or consider sharing one with a friend. Half the pudding equals half the calories.
- Once you begin to feel satisfied, stop eating. Listen to your body and what it tells you. Don't keep eating until you feel stuffed. You can always take the remaining portions home with you.
- Remember that it's okay to choose your favorite foods now and then, even if you consider them 'not-so-healthy.' You shouldn't continuously deprive yourself of

foods you truly love, even when eating out. As long as you eat them in moderation and know when to stop, a few treats here and there can still be a part of a healthy diet and lifestyle!

Most of all, remember who is in charge of what goes in your mouth. Ask what's in various dishes, and think of the menu as only a small selection of what's available. For example, if you like the sound of the fish but not the cream sauce, ask for it without the sauce or request another method of cooking. The rule of thumb in any restaurant is to choose something simple without a sauce that contains unknown ingredients. You can't go wrong with grilled fish or chicken served with vegetables or a salad.

HITTING A WEIGHT-LOSS PLATEAU

In the first few weeks of the Lemon Juice Diet you will probably notice a weight loss of around seven pounds. In the weeks after that, some of you may find that the weight doesn't fall off so fast, even though you are exercising regularly and eating healthily.

When weight plateaus, often you are actually closer than ever to losing weight. However, seeing your weight stay the same for weeks on end after an initial weight loss is a natural and common occurrence caused by your body's instinctive need to maintain equilibrium. Once your body has got used to a new routine of eating and exercising, it gradually adjusts its metabolism to safeguard its fat reserves. It's at this point that you'll notice your eating and exercise efforts aren't producing the same weight-loss results as before, and the needle on the scales sits stubbornly in the same place.

If you still have weight to lose it is important to keep eating healthily when your weight loss plateaus. Trying to speed up weight loss by severely restricting your food intake is no solution – your body will recognize the reduction in calories and cling to fat ever harder. Don't get angry with yourself either. Instead, think of how far you have come and how much weight you have lost. Think about how much better you feel now that you are eating healthily and how much easier it is to climb stairs or run after the children. Make a mental note of all the improvements you notice to help you stay motivated.

Is this Really a Plateau?

If you want to weigh yourself, bear in mind that your weight can fluctuate throughout the day due to many factors, such as food consumption and water retention. Though there is no best time of day to weigh yourself, experts suggest you pick the same time every week and use the same scales. Check your weight no more than once or perhaps twice a week – any more frequently and you may get discouraged by normal fluctuations in your reading. Also, be consistent in what you wear when weighing in. Remember too that muscle weighs more than fat so that the numbers on the scales can be misleading. Other indicators, such as body fat percentage, readings from a tape measure and how well you fit into your clothes should be taken into account as well.

If you've been eating healthily and exercising regularly and your weight has hit a plateau for several months, then you need to think about whether this is really a plateau, or whether you have indeed reached your natural weight or the weight at which your body feels comfortable. If you are 30 pounds over what is ideal for your height and build, this could be a plateau, but if you are just 5 or even 10 pounds away, you might consider accepting your weight. Is it really worth punishing your body with a strict regime to achieve a weight that is perhaps unnatural and unhealthy for you?

If you are doing any strength training or muscle work, scales can be misleading because muscles weigh more than fat. You may not show a weight loss, but with muscle replacing fat you will look a lot better.

It might be worth having a check-up with your doctor to see if you have any condition that interferes with weight loss, such as diabetes, PCOS, thyroid problems or other hormonal imbalance. It is also important to consider where your fat is stored. If it's stored around your middle, this poses the greatest risk to your health. Fat stores accumulated here are associated with heart disease, diabetes and even cancer.

If you really feel you have reached a plateau and that you do need to lose some more weight, there are two things you can do to promote weight loss: modify your eating habits and change your exercise program in a way that challenges your body.

Start with Your Diet

Are You Drinking Enough?

As you saw in the Lemon Juice Diet principles in Chapter 4, drinking plenty of water is essential to weight loss, since burning fat increases the toxins in your system that then need to be flushed out by your liver and kidneys. If there isn't adequate water to do this, your body will burn fat less effi- ciently as this natural function won't be triggered. If you're eating properly and exercising regularly at a high intensity, increasing your water intake may be just the thing you need to get your weight loss back on track. You should drink up to 3½ pints a day (or more if it's hot or you are exercising), and cut back on coffee, tea or other drinks that may dehydrate you. Drinking more than one glass of lemon juice a day will also help.

Review Your Food Diary

Sometimes, when you start to lose weight, you are not as diligent as you were at the beginning of the diet. Portion sizes start to increase. Sweets creep back into your diet. You could be eating more calories than you think. These are further reasons why keeping a food diary and recording everything you eat is a good idea. It can help you see what might be holding you back from further weight loss. This doesn't mean you have to restrict your diet severely. It just means making a few small changes, such as eating more fruit, having a salad a day, and avoiding high-calorie foods.

Forgive Yourself

Many people have an 'all or nothing' way of thinking when it comes to healthy eating. They feel guilty or angry with themselves when they lapse, and then carry on eating poorly because of these negative feelings. The first step is to forgive yourself: what you've eaten isn't the problem, but how you've reacted to it is. If you've lapsed recently, remind yourself that no one is perfect and tomorrow is another day.

Ask for Help

Social support from a partner, slimming group, friend or website can provide essential help and emotional encouragement. And statistics show that people who have a support system tend to lose weight and keep it off, as they can share their diet ups and downs with others.

Slow Down

Many people have unrealistic weight-loss goals. When you start eating healthily, and combine this with regular exercise, you will lose a lot of weight – but most of this is water. After losing this initial weight, people tend to lose one pound a week on average, which is still considered good progress (even a few pounds a month is good). In fact, slow but steady is the best way to lose weight because studies show that people who lose weight slowly and gradually at a rate of one or two pounds a week tend to be most successful at losing weight and keeping it off.

Look Beyond Your Diet

Are other factors getting in the way of your weight-loss efforts? For example, stress might be bringing up inner feelings and needs that are sabotaging your eating plan. Go back to your food diary and jot down the thoughts and feelings that make you want to eat, or use your social support network to talk about the emotional connection between food and mood.

Be Prepared

Always eat breakfast so you don't start the day feeling hungry, and make sure your environment complements your diet. This might mean taking healthy snacks to work with you, or filling your fridge with healthy foods so you're not tempted to eat things that might sabotage your diet.

Eat Little and Often

Don't forget the importance of eating small meals frequently for weight loss. The little-and-often approach can help regulate your blood sugar and appetite. Also, as your body expends energy when digesting food, eating several mini-meals a day can help boost your metabolism.

Review Your Exercise Routine

Now that you know what kind of changes you need to make to your diet to start losing weight again, you can focus on subtly modifying your exercise routine to get the results you want.

Consider Cross-training
Are you stuck in an exercise rut? Running the same number of miles a week? Swimming the same number of lengths? When muscles get used to an exercise pattern, they begin to adapt, and your body burns fewer calories doing it. To keep your calorie burn high, mix your workouts. Combine walking with cycling, jogging with swimming or stair-climbing with aerobics, and so on.

Increase the Intensity
If you are exercising aerobically, it might be time to increase the length or intensity of your workout. Studies have shown that exercising for 45 minutes five times a week is effective for weight loss, but if you haven't got the time to spare, intensify your workouts by making your movements more precise and not resting between moves. There's no need to increase the duration of your workout – just your effort.

You could build up the intensity of your workout by picking up the pace for one to three minutes, then returning to your normal pace for three to five minutes. Repeat this cycle throughout your workout as it will help you burn more calories.

Exercise First Thing
If you can, try to exercise first thing in the morning as this will kick-start your metabolism and help you burn fat stores all day. If you aren't used to morning exercise, make sure you have a light snack such as a piece of fruit and a dry biscuit before you begin; then have your breakfast after your workout.

Get Pumped

Are you doing enough strength training? Muscles require more energy to function than fat does, so if you increase your muscle mass you'll raise the speed at which you burn calories and, consequently, fat. Women often lose weight by cutting calories and only doing aerobic exercise such as walking, but this means they lose muscle along with fat, and each pound of muscle you lose decreases the amount you must eat to maintain your weight by 35 calories. The secret is to maximize fat loss while maintaining muscle tone. Keep doing aerobic activity but start to do weight training or muscle toning exercises for a slimmer, firmer body. Remember that with weight training you must ensure you have a rest day between sessions.

Are You Active Enough?

Think about how active you are in your daily life. In this age of internet shopping, phones, email, cars, elevators and televisions, we are far less active than our parents were 50 years ago. Try to keep as active as possible during the day.

Have a Rest

During exercise you stress your system, and if you don't allow your body to recuperate adequately between sessions, you can actually lose muscle tissue. This, in turn, will cause your metabolism to slow down. Allowing your muscles to recover, along with following a proper diet, is ultimately what makes you more toned and sculpted. Also, by letting your body recover properly, you can work to maximum capacity in your next workout and so burn more fat. So, if you are exercising more than five days a week or for more than two hours a day, it may be time to cut back.

Once you have fine-tuned your diet and workout program, you should start to notice a difference in how you look in the weeks ahead. Above all, be patient with yourself. If you keep eating healthily, exercising regularly and enjoying your life, your body will eventually settle at a weight that is perfect for you.

THINK POSITIVE

Just remember that a huge part of looking and feeling great is about the way you think of yourself – and weight loss begins in your head. To lose weight successfully you have to change your attitudes and your thoughts about food and yourself. You need to start seeing food not as the enemy but as a wonderful source of nutrients that can give you energy and help you lose weight. You have to start seeing yourself as a person who is in control of their life, not as someone who lets things happen to them.

The motivation to lose weight has to come from within. Attitude is everything. The very fact that you have read this far shows that you are highly motivated to lose weight; all you need to do now is give up negative self-belief. Changing negative beliefs is vital for success on the Lemon Juice Diet. If you think you're fat or lacking in willpower, addicted to junk food or can't ever lose weight, you're probably right; but you can change your mind if you want to, and when you change your mind, your body will follow.

Although there will be setbacks along the way, if you stay positive and clearheaded you stack the odds in your favor. For example, instead of thinking about the weight you need to lose, think about how much slimmer, fitter, and healthier you want to feel. Instead of giving up when you succumb to temptation, rise to the occasion or simply get back to your healthy eating plan.

Having a positive image of yourself and your ability to cope with setbacks is the first step on the road to being slimmer but by itself it isn't enough. Positive expectation is the second step and taking action is the third. It's no good hoping you will succeed; you need to take responsibility for your life, believe you can succeed and make positive changes. In other words, you need to direct both your thoughts and your actions to achieving your weight-loss goal.

Thinking isn't enough; it's the doing that counts. And this is where you stop thinking about the Lemon Juice Diet and start doing it! This is where you stop wishing you could lose weight and start losing it!

Fourteen Golden Tips

1. Start your day with a glass of fresh lemon juice.
2. Always eat breakfast.
3. Keep your blood sugar levels balanced with three meals a day based on whole, unrefined foods with two healthy snacks such as fresh fruit and nuts in between.
4. Eat fresh whole foods, preferably organic.
5. Eat plenty of vegetables and fruit.
6. Eat some quality protein with every meal.
7. Get your essential fats.
8. Drink plenty of water.
9. Reduce your intake of caffeine, alcohol and saturated fat.
10. Read food labels and avoid food rich in additives and preservatives.
11. Chew your food and take your time over meals.
12. Pass on the sugar, the meat, the dairy and the salt.
13. Use lemon juice in your cooking and to sprinkle over your meals.
14. Get moving for at least 30 minutes a day.

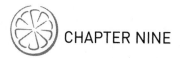 CHAPTER NINE

Lemon Cures

Lemons have been used for centuries to treat a variety of health concerns. For instance, many Ancient Egyptians believed that eating lemons and drinking lemon juice was an effective protection against a variety of poisons, and recent research has confirmed this belief.

As well as improving your digestion and helping you shed pounds, lemons have been shown to have antibacterial, antiviral and immune-boosting powers. A strong immune system is essential for good overall health, and lemons can help to stimulate your body's immune system and reduce the risk of illness – in the most natural way possible. This is because they contain many substances that promote immunity and fight infection, notably citric acid, calcium, magnesium, vitamin C, bioflavonoids, pectin and limonene. So whenever you feel that your immune system needs a boost, try drinking a few glasses of lemon juice diluted with water or eating a raw lemon.

Lemons and lemon-scented plants (*see box below*) can be used internally and externally for a huge range of purposes. In this chapter you will find suggestions for using lemons to treat a variety of conditions. Whether you use them in the form of juices, teas, drinks, dressings, poultices or in the bath, take advantage of their natural power to heal.

Lemon-Scented Plants

Lemongrass: A Southeast Asian plant from the liquorice family. It has a lemony flavor when chewed and contains healing essential oils. Teas prepared with lemongrass are used to treat digestive complaints. Externally, the oils can soothe muscular pain. The healing powers of lemongrass are often used in combination with lemon itself. To make lemon grass tea, you will need: 2 tsp dried lemongrass, 250 ml/ 9 fl oz hot water, 1 tbsp freshly squeezed lemon juice and maple syrup to taste. Pour hot water over the lemongrass and let it seep for 10 minutes. Pour through a sieve and add the lemon juice and maple syrup.

Lemon Pelargonium: These fragrant plants are used to add lemon aroma to baked goods or sweets. For potpourri and as indoor plants they are thought to neutralize the smell of cigarette smoke. Of the many pelargonium plants, the 'Queen of Lemon' has the most pungent lemon smell.

> Lemon Balm: Lemon balm contains Melissa oil and, like lemongrass, is unrelated to the lemon plant. Lemon balm tea is a proven tonic for insomnia and anxiety. When combined with the substances in lemons that are known to stimulate immunity, it is also soothing and healing for colds, influenza, headaches and respiratory inflammations.

Acne

Lemons contain citric acid, which can be effective in treating acne and drying out spots. The vitamin C found in citrus fruit is vital for healthy, glowing skin, while its alkaline nature kills some types of bacteria known to cause acne. In addition to drinking lemon juice with water first thing in the morning, here are some suggestions for homemade acne treatments.

- Apply fresh lemon juice to the acne and leave overnight. Wash with water the following morning. You can squeeze some lemon juice onto your finger or a cotton ball and apply it directly to the skin. There may be an uncomfortable burning sensation at first but this will soon disappear.
- Mix one part of freshly squeezed lemon juice with an equal part of rose or honey water. Apply the mixture to

the affected areas and leave for at least half an hour, then wash with water. This application should be repeated twice daily, ideally in the morning and the evening.

These remedies are natural and safe but if acne is severe or there are open wounds, it is always best to consult your doctor first.

Anxiety

Research has shown that lemon balm has a calming effect and therefore may be able to help fatigue, exhaustion, dizziness, anxiety, nervousness and nervous tension. It has the ability to refresh the mind by creating a positive outlook and removing negative emotions. It is also believed that inhaling lemon oil helps increase concentration and alertness so it can be effective as a room freshener in offices to improve efficiency. If you're feeling tense, sprinkle a few drops of lemon balm (melissa) on a handkerchief to inhale.

Bloating

Lemon juice diluted with water and drunk daily on an empty stomach first thing in the morning can help eliminate water retention.

Cankers (mouth ulcers)

The proven antibacterial and antiviral properties of lemons can accelerate the healing process in the case of cankers. Mix the juice of a freshly squeezed lemon into a glass of lukewarm water and rinse your mouth with this solution; do this three times a day. There may be a burning sensation when the lemon juice comes into contact with the canker, but the more frequently you use it the less burning there will be. Remember, don't brush your teeth after rinsing with lemon juice; wait at least half an hour.

Cellulite

Lemon essential oil has tissue-strengthening properties that may help restore the weakened connective tissue that triggers cellulite. Simply mix a few drops of lemon essential oil with 1 tbsp jojoba oil and massage the areas affected by cellulite morning and evening.

Chills and Fevers

Here is a method that can ease symptoms: add the juice of one lemon to a cup of hot water with honey and drink at once, then every two hours till the fever or chill subsides.

Cold Sores

The antiviral properties of lemon can help heal cold sores. Place a drop of undiluted lemon essential oil on the end of a cotton swab and dab onto the cold sore. Do not make any brushing or stroking movements because if the blister breaks this will spread the infection. At the same time, boost your immune system by drinking two or three glasses of diluted lemon juice a day.

Colds

During a cold the healing power of lemons works internally by supplying urgently required vitamin C to the defense cells. Meanwhile, its antiviral properties get to work on the virus on the mucous membranes in the nose and throat.

At the first indication of a cold – a runny nose or sore throat – you should try to give your body as much immune-boosting vitamin C as you can to eliminate the virus before it gets a chance to take hold. Drink the freshly squeezed juice of one lemon in a glass of lukewarm water every two hours.

If you have a sore throat, add the juice of a lemon and 1 tsp sea salt to 9 fl oz lukewarm water. Gargle three times a day for a minute to diminish the burning sensation. If it's a case of tonsillitis, gargle every two hours for at least 30 seconds with the freshly squeezed juice of a lemon. Tilt your head back to allow the antibacterial and antiviral properties of the juice to flow into the back of the throat. You can swallow the juice when you have finished gargling, thereby benefiting from an immune-boosting shot of vitamin C.

Corns

Lemon poultices applied overnight are a good home remedy for corns and calluses. Place a slice of lemon about ¼ inch thick onto the corn; bandage and fasten. Dabbing the affected area with lemon essential oil also helps accelerate the healing process. Take care to use the undiluted oil only on the callused area using a cotton ball or cotton swab.

Diarrhea

Lemon juice has proven itself as a disinfectant against cholera bacteria and is an excellent treatment for diarrhea. If you get a bout of diarrhea, drink the juice of a freshly squeezed lemon in a large glass of water three times a day. As a preventive measure, take 1–2 tbsp lemon juice before every meal.

Eczema

If you suffer from skin infection a lemon wrap may offer relief. Add eight drops of lemon essential oil to 9 fl oz lukewarm water and 1 tbsp liquid honey. (Honey also has anti-inflammatory effects and strengthens the healing power of lemon.) Soak a linen cloth in the liquid, squeeze out excess fluid and gently place the cloth on the affected area for 15 minutes, two or three times a day. Not only will this ease the infection, it will also counter the overwhelming urge to scratch.

Pure lemon juice can also help heal minor skin infections. Just place a few drops directly on to the affected area and gently spread it. There may be a slight burning sensation in the first few minutes.

Fatigue

Long-distance walkers as well as world travelers and explorers look upon the lemon as a godsend. When fatigue begins to set in, a lemon is sucked through a hole in the top. This provides quick refreshment, as a small amount of lemon juice will quench thirst more effectively than many times the amount of water. Explorers use lemon for protection against many tropical infections. Experienced travelers add lemon juice to ordinary drinking water because it acts as an antiseptic and prevents illness.

Lemon oil also seems to be able to stimulate brain activity, so whenever you feel tired for no reason or are finding it hard to focus or concentrate, add four drops of lemon oil to a water-filled aromatherapy lamp. Alternatively, drink a glass of lemon water every few hours.

Gout

Lemon juice is proven to help prevent gout attacks because it helps stimulate the formation of calcium carbonate in the body. This substance neutralizes acids, especially uric acid which triggers gout. After each main meal, drink the freshly squeezed juice of a lemon in a glass of lukewarm water.

Gum Disease

To prevent or treat gum disease, pour the freshly squeezed juice of one lemon into a glass of lukewarm water. Take a mouthful and rinse for a minute; the lemon juice will help kill the bacteria and the acid will help dissolve the plaque. Wait at least half an hour before brushing your teeth.

Halitosis (bad breath)

Lemons can help freshen breath that has gone sour after eating certain spices, drinking alcohol, smoking cigarettes or because of insufficient salivation. To keep breath fresh, thoroughly rinse your mouth several times a day with the freshly squeezed juice of a lemon in a glass of lukewarm water. Chewing on a lemon slice after every meal will also help. Wait at least half an hour before brushing your teeth after chewing or rinsing with lemon juice.

High Blood Pressure

Garlic and onions have been shown to be effective in the fight against high blood pressure, and combine well with the healing power of lemon. Add three crushed garlic cloves and one chopped onion to 1¾ pints of cold skimmed, low-fat or soya milk. Slowly bring to the boil and let it stand for five minutes. Pour through a sieve and chill. Add the freshly squeezed juice of three lemons and sip throughout the day.

High Cholesterol
The pectin power in lemons, along with their other metabolism- and circulation-boosting nutrients, can help lower cholesterol.

Insect Bites
If a wasp stinger is still in the skin take it out with a pair of tweezers. Massage one or two drops of lemon essential oil mixed with 1 tsp honey into the skin around the bite.

To repel insects add 20 drops of lemon oil to 9 fl oz water and spray into the air. It smells great too. Another home remedy is to place a cotton ball soaked in lemon essential oil in your bedroom. If you are sitting outside in the evening, apply lemon scent to skin areas not covered by clothing. Add 10 drops of lemon essential oil to 4 tbsp (2 fl oz) sunflower oil and rub into the skin.

Insomnia
Several studies have found that lemon balm combined with other calming herbs (such as valerian, hops, and chamomile) helps reduce anxiety and promote sleep. In a recent study, 18 healthy volunteers received two separate single doses of a standardized lemon balm extract (300 mg and 600 mg) or a placebo for seven days. The 600 mg dose of lemon balm was found to elevate mood and significantly increase calmness and alertness.

Lemon balm is available as a dried leaf that can be bought in bulk. It is also sold as tea, and in capsules, extracts, tinctures and oil. For difficulty in sleeping (or to reduce stomach complaints, flatulence, or bloating) choose from the following:

Tea: Steep ¼–1 tsp dried lemon balm herb in hot water. Drink up to four times daily

Tincture: Take 40–90 drops three times daily

Capsules: Take 300–500 mg dried lemon balm three times daily, or as needed

Nosebleeds

Squeeze some juice from a fresh lemon, soak a cotton swab in it and dab the inside of the nose gently. Lemons have astringent properties and as soon as injured blood vessels come into contact with the juice they contract and the wound starts to close.

Rheumatism

Even though it tastes bitter, lemon juice has a powerful alkaline effect in the body. It is therefore a natural agent against excess acid, which is partly responsible for rheumatism. Drink the freshly squeezed juice of a lemon in a glass of lukewarm water three times a day. If you experience severe pain add the juice of two lemons three times a day.

Lemon essential oil has pain-relieving qualities so to inhibit inflammation and ease pain you may want to massage the affected area daily with several drops of lemon oil mixed with 1 tbsp jojoba oil.

Stomach Upsets
Drink the juice of a freshly squeezed lemon in a glass of lukewarm water after each meal. The lemon juice will stimulate the production of stomach acid and the activity of stomach muscles.

Vaginal Hygiene
It is safe to wash the vaginal area in diluted lemon juice. Although it is a powerful antiseptic it is nevertheless free from irritating drugs often found in douches and pessaries. Its proven antibacterial qualities suggest that it may be able to boost immunity and ward off infection.

Varicose and Spider Veins
Lemon essential oil has vessel-strengthening properties that can help fight varicose and spider veins.

🍋 For spider veins, mix two or three drops of lemon oil in a small bowl with 3 tbsp (1½ fl oz) jojoba, avocado, or almond oil. Massage the affected area every day.

- For varicose veins, add six drops of lemon oil to 4 tbsp (2 fl oz) wheat germ oil, and two drops each of cypress and juniper oil. Use this mixture daily for a gentle massage of the legs from bottom to top in the direction of the heart.
- For a vein and vessel rejuvenating bath, add eight drops of lemon oil to warm bath water. Also, add four drops of cypress oil blended with 1 tbsp liquid honey. Soak in the bath for 15 minutes and pat, don't rub, your skin dry.

REFERENCES

Diets Don't Work

Mann, T. et al. 'Medicare's Search for Effective Obesity Treatments: Diets Are Not the Answer', *Am. Psychol.*, 2007 Apr; 62(3):220–33

http://www.senseaboutscience.org.uk/index.php/site/project/47

Importance of Good Digestion for Health and Weight Loss

Blaut, T. et al. 'Metabolic diversity of the intestinal microbiota: implications for health and disease', *J. Nutr.*, 2007 Mar; 137(3 Suppl. 2):751S–5S

Had, B. et al. 'Intestinal gas production from bacterial fermentation of undigested carbohydrate in irritable bowel syndrome', *Am. J. Gastroenterol.*, 1989 Apr; 84(4):375–8

Spiller, R. et al. 'Guidelines for the management of Irritable Bowel Syndrome', *Gut*, 2007 May 8

Cayenne Pepper and Metabolism

Ahuja, D. et al. 'Effects of chili consumption on postprandial glucose, insulin, and energy metabolism', *Am. J. Clin. Nutr.*, 2006 Jul; 84(1):63–9

Importance of Nutritional Detoxification

Crinnion, W. 'Environmental Medicine, Part 1: The Human Burden of Environmental Toxins and Their Common Health Effects', *Alt. Med. Rev.*, 2000, 5(1), 52–63

Kidd, P.M. 'Glutathione: Systemic Protectant Against Oxidative and Free Radical Damage', *Alt. Med. Rev.*, 1997, 2(3):155–176

Parke, D. et al. 'Nutritional requirements for detoxication of environmental chemicals', *Food Addit. Contam.*, 1991 May–Jun; 8(3):381–96

Pool, B. et al. 'Modulation of xenobiotic metabolising enzymes by anticarcinogens – focus on glutathione S-transferases and their role as targets of dietary chemoprevention in colorectal carcinogenesis', *Mutation Research*, 2005 Dec 11; 591(1–2):74–92. Epub 2005 Aug 3

Lemon as a Digestive Aid

(No authors listed) 'Lemonade blocks kidney stone formation', *Health News*, 2006 Aug; 12(8):10–11

Baghurst, Dr. Katrine. *The Health Benefits of Citrus Fruits* (2003), Consumer Science Program, CSIRO Health Sciences & Nutrition; www.austcitrus.org.au

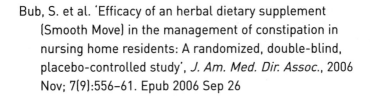

Bub, S. et al. 'Efficacy of an herbal dietary supplement (Smooth Move) in the management of constipation in nursing home residents: A randomized, double-blind, placebo-controlled study', *J. Am. Med. Dir. Assoc.*, 2006 Nov; 7(9):556–61. Epub 2006 Sep 26

Cherng, S.C. et al. 'Acceleration of hepatobiliary excretion by lemon juice on 99mTc-tetrofosmin cardiac SPECT', *Nucl. Med. Commun.*, 2006 Nov; 27(11):859–64

de Castillo, M.C. et al. 'Bactericidal activity of lemon juice and lemon derivatives against Vibrio cholerae', *Pharm. Bull.*, 2000 Oct; 23(10):1235–8

Deyhim, F. et al. 'Citrus juice modulates antioxidant enzymes and lipid profiles in orchidectomized rats', *J. Med. Food*, 2006 Fall; 9(3):422–6

Grassmann, J. et al. 'Antioxidative effects of lemon oil and its components on copper induced oxidation of low density lipoprotein', *Arzneimittelforschung*, 2001 Oct; 51(10):799–805

Kang, D.E. et al. 'Long-term lemonade based dietary manipulation in patients with hypocitraturic nephrolithiasis', *J. Urol.*, 2007 Apr; 177(4):1358–62

Olivares, M. et al. 'Iron absorption from wheat flour: effects of lemonade and chamomile infusion', *Nutrition*, 2007 Apr; 23(4):296–300. Epub 2007 Mar 13

Ostman, E. 'Vinegar supplementation lowers glucose and insulin responses and increases satiety after a bread meal in healthy subjects', *Eur. J. Clin. Nutr.*, 2005 Sep; 59(9):983–8

Lemon as a Liver Tonic
Rapavi, E. et al. 'The effect of citrus flavonoids on the redox state of alimentary-induced fatty liver in rats', *Nat. Prod. Res.*, 2007 Mar; 21(3):274–81

Tirkey, N. et al. 'Hesperidin, a citrus bioflavonoid, decreases the oxidative stress produced by carbon tetrachloride in rat liver and kidney', *BMC Pharmacol.*, 2005 Jan 31; 5(1):2

Lemons and Stress
(No authors listed) 'Lemon oil vapour causes an anti-stress effect via modulating the 5-HT and DA activities in mice', PubMed.gov., (2006-06-15)

Cerny, A. et al. 'Tolerability and efficacy of valerian/lemon balm in healthy volunteers (a double-blind, placebo-controlled, multicentre study)', *Fitoterapia*, 1999; 70:221–228

de Sousa, A.C. et al. 'Melissa officinalis L. essential oil: antitumoral and antioxidant activities', *J. Pharm. Pharmacol.*, 2004; 56(5):677–81

Limonene

Chow, S. et al. 'Pharmacokinetics of Perillic Acid in Humans after a Single Dose Administration of a Citrus Preparation Rich in d-limonene Content', *Cancer Epidemiology, Biomarkers & Prevention*, 2002; 11:1472–1476

Elson, C.E. et al. 'Anti-carcinogenic activity of d-limonene during the initiation and promotion/progression stages of DMBA-induced rat mammary carcinogenesis', *Carcinogenesis*, 1998; 9:331–332

Lu, X.G. et al. 'Inhibition of growth and metastasis of human gastric cancer implanted in nude mice by d-limonene', *World J. Gastroenterol.*, 2004 Jul 15; 10(14):2140–4

Maltzman, T.H. 'The prevention of nitosomethylurea-induced mammary tumors by d-limonene and orange oil', *Carcinogenesis*, 1989; 10:781–783

Wattenberg, L.W. et al. 'Inhibition of 4-(methylnitrosoamino)-1-(3-pyridyl)-1-butanone carcinogenesis in mice by d-limonene and citrus fruit oils', *Carcinogenesis*, 1991; 12:115–117

Yano, H. et al. 'Attenuation of d-limonene of sodium chloride-enhanced gastric carcinogenesis induced by N-methyl-N-nitro-N-nitrosoguanidine in Wistar rats', *International Journal of Cancer*, 1999; 8:665–668

Liver Dysfunction and Obesity
Brunt, E. et al. 'Pathology of fatty liver disease', *Mod. Pathol.*, 2007 Feb; 20 Suppl 1:S40–8

Pectin and Hunger
Delargy, J. et al. 'Effects of amount and type of dietary fibre (soluble and insoluble) on short-term control of appetite', *Int. J. Food Sci. Nutr.*, 1997 Jan; 48(1):67–77

pH Balance
Rapavi, E. et al. 'Effects of citrus flavonoids on redox homeostasis of toxin-injured liver in rat', *Acta. Biol. Hung.*, 2006 Dec; 57(4):415–22

Quercetin and Insulin
Kanter, M. et al. 'The effects of quercetin on bone minerals, biomechanical behavior, and structure in streptozotocin-induced diabetic rats', *Cell. Biochem. Funct.*, 2007 Jan 31

Vitamin C and Weight Loss
Johnston, C. et al. 'Strategies for healthy weight loss: from vitamin C to the glycemic response', *J. Am. Coll. Nutr.*, 2005 Jun; 24(3):158–65

Calcium and Weight Loss

Kabmova, K. et al. 'Calcium intake and the outcome of short-term weight management', *Physiol. Res.*, 2007 May 30

Lemon: Healing and Immune-boosting Properties

(No authors listed) 'Antibacterial activity of citrus fruit juices against Vibrio species', *J. Nutr. Sci. Vitaminol.* (Tokyo), 2006 Apr; 52(2):157–60

Baghurst, Dr. Katrine. Op cit.

Berhow, M.A. et al. 'Acylated flavonoids in callus cultures of Citrus aurantifolia', *Phytochemistry*, 1994 Jul; 36(5):1225–7

de Castillo, M. et al. Op. cit.

Gharagozloo, M. et al. 'Immunomodulatory effect of concentrated lime juice extract on activated human mononuclear cells', *J. Ethnopharmacol.*, 2001 Sep; 77(1):85–90

Grassmann, J. et al. 'Antioxidative effects of lemon oil and its components on copper induced oxidation of low density lipoprotein', *Arzneimittelforschung*, 2001 Oct; 51(10):799–805

Joshipura, K.J. et al. 'The effect of fruit and vegetable intake on risk of coronary heart disease', *Annals Int. Med.*, 2001

Jung, U. et al. 'Effect of citrus flavonoids on lipid metabolism and glucose-regulating enzyme mRNA levels in type-2 diabetic mice', *Int. J. Biochem. Cell Biol.*, 2006; 38(7):1134–45. Epub 2006 Jan 6

Kawaii, S. et al. 'Antiproliferative effects of the readily extractable fractions prepared from various citrus juices on several cancer cell lines', *J. Agric. Food Chem.*, 1999 Jul; 47(7):2509–12

Khaw, K. et al. 'Relation between plasma ascorbic acid and mortality in men and women in EPIC-Norfolk prospective study: a prospective population study', European Prospective Investigation into Cancer and Nutrition, *Lancet*, 2001 Mar 3; 357(9257):657–63

Kurl, S. et al. 'Plasma vitamin C modifies the association between hypertension and risk of stroke', *Stroke*, 2002 Jun; 33(6):1568–73

Lu, X.G. et al. Op. cit.

Misra, N. et al. Fungitoxic properties of the essential oil of Citrus limon (L.) Burm. against a few dermatophytes', *Mycoses*, 1988 Jul; 31(7):380–2

Miyake, Y. et al. 'Identification of coumarins from lemon fruit (Citrus limon) as inhibitors of in vitro tumor promotion and superoxide and nitric oxide generation', *J. Agric. Food Chem.*, 1999 Aug; 47(8):3151–7

Ogata, S. et al. 'Apoptosis induced by the flavonoid from lemon fruit (Citrus limon BURM. f.) and its metabolites in HL-60 cells', *Biosci. Biotechnol. Biochem.*, 2000 May; 64(5):1075-8

Rodrigues, A. et al. 'Protection from cholera by adding lemon juice to food – results from community and laboratory studies in Guinea-Bissau, West Africa', *Trop. Med. Int. Health*, 2000 Jun; 5(6):418–22

Wood, M. 'Citrus Compound, Ready to Help Your Body!', *Agricultural Research*, February 2005

Index